SPEECHLESS

My Recovery from Stroke

by JENNIFER GORDON

First published in 1994 by
University of Western Australia Press
Nedlands, Western Australia 6009

This book is copyright, Apart from any fair dealing for the purpose of private study, research, criticism or review, as permitted under the Copyright Act 1968, no part may be reproduced by any process without written permission. Enquiries should be made to the publisher.

© Jennifer Gordon 1994

Editions: 1st print 1994; 2nd print 2011

National Library of Australia
Cataloguing-in-Publication entry:

Gordon, Jennifer, 1945-
    Speechless

ISBN 978-0-646-55682-6
1. Gordon, Jennifer, 1945- — Health. 2. Cerebrovascular disease — Patients — Biography. 3. Cerebrovascular disease —
— Patients — Rehabilitation. 4. Speech disorders. 1. Title

362.196810092

Cover image: *'Collage - representing my way of thinking at that time'*, and drawings *by* Jennifer Gordon

Printed by Gateway Printing, Perth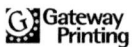

FOR BENJAMIN AND AMANDA
WITH ALL MY LOVE

FOREWORD

To communicate is as fundamental to an independent existence as it is to be human. *Speechless* is a story recounted by an intelligent, brave and resourceful woman who abruptly and selectively lost her ability both to speak and to communicate. The ischaemic stroke she suffered injured the left frontal cortex of her brain. Non-verbal emotional expression, including gesture, was also lost, resulting in situations that were at the same time amusing and tragic and yet extremely informative. Although she retained the ability to write, she was unable to select the appropriate words or to use them to construct sentences. Later, after some recovery, the impaired orchestration of an emotional framework for the use of words continued to severely restrict her independence.

The struggle to regain her use of language is dramatically illustrated by the description of her experiences with hospital staff, therapists, doctors, shop assistants, employers, friends and family. Above all, her recall of the features considered by her to be important during this recovery process, particularly the 'brain clicks', makes compelling reading in the genre of Luria's *The Man With a Shattered World*.

That someone so devastatingly incapacitated, yet outwardly unaffected, could subsequently produce such an informative and amusing account of her experience is a remarkable testimony to her fortitude and to the power of the recovery process contained within the human brain.

Dr W.M. Carroll, MB, BS,MD,FRACP
Consultant Neurologist
Head of Neurology Department
Queen Elizabeth 11 Medical Centre
Perth, Western Australia

PREFACE

About five weeks after the stroke, I managed to convey to friends that I would like to read a book about the experiences of a 'speech stroke' patient so that I could see how the author coped. But they were unable to find one. I became convinced that I should write about my experiences myself, when I was able. Since finishing the book, I have discovered there are a few books on the topic of 'speech stroke'; I have included these in my Further Reading listing.

I finally started to write the book eighteen months after the stroke and it took me a further eighteen months to complete (mid-1991). Dr Rosemary German-Belmont, Vonny Johnson, and Yvonne Bryce read the first pages – and their surprise was too great to be feigned: 'I never guessed you were thinking this...'. Reassured by their enthusiasm, I hastened to produce more pages.

Margaret MacPherson and I spent a weekend at Fairbridge Farm at Pinjarra, south of Perth, where we sat up far into the night tweaking the final version.

I feel it should be noted that all the symptoms I describe in Chapter One may not necessarily be the symptoms of stroke. Some of them may just reflect my state of health at the time. But the neurological symptoms listed in this chapter do indicate the possible onset of stroke. There is also a difference of medical opinion about prolonged stress as a factor in stroke.

Jennifer Gordon
April 1994

PREFACE TO THE SECOND EDITION

I have left the main text of the book largely unchanged and added a short chapter to show a brief glimpse of life at twenty-three years further on. As well, I have changed the cover and added pictures, which I drew shortly after the stroke.

I sincerely hope that all those people who read my book and those who did not are well, happy and leading fulfilling lives, as I am.

Jennifer Gordon
April 2011

ACKNOWLEDGEMENTS

My sincere thanks to all those people, mentioned in this book, who gave me endless encouragement and who stayed my friends throughout the course of the stroke. These people stood by me in spite of my inability to tell them what I was thinking and feeling and were still there when I finally recovered enough to write about my experiences. I am especially grateful to my resourceful son, Dr Benjamin Gordon, and my good friend Dr Rosemary German-Belmont.

My grateful thanks go to Shauna Forrest, Kathryn Hird, Chris Smith, Suzanne Humphries, Isobel Currie and Jan Zach, my speech pathologists, for their endless patience and great good humour. I attend a group session with my speech pathologist and friend, Melita Brown and I am still improving more than I thought possible at this stage, nearly six years after the stroke. Some health professionals were of the opinion there would be very little improvement after two years.

I thank, with all my heart, my good friends at South Perth Community Hospital where I worked as a kitchen assistant: Sandra Feld, Rod Brown and Wilhelmina Fernandez (the cooks) and all the 'girls'. They managed to turn a blind eye to my mistakes, which did so much for my self-esteem and hastened my recovery. In particular, warm thanks must go to Peter Aylmore for his lively sense of malice coupled uncomfortably to a heart of gold.

I owe a special debt of gratitude to the late Colleen McIntosh, Director of Nursing, who took a chance on me and who was unfailingly kind to me.

I am indebted to Dr Brendan Kay, who looked after my precious dog Maggie and cat Hiraeth. And to my neighbour

Terry Tyak for looking after my house and cat while I was in hospital.

Many thanks to my proof-readers – Dr Benjamin Gordon, Michael Crouch, Dr W.M Carroll, Margaret MacPherson, Professor Allen German and Rod Brown - for their interest, encouragement and sound advice.

I would like to acknowledge and thank my editor, Amanda Curtin, for her tactful and sensitive assistance in improving the quality of the text. And Janine and Ian Drakeford of the University of Western Australia Press, responsible for the book's first publication in 1994.

Finally to Dr W.M. Carroll, specialist neurologist, my grateful thanks to him for writing the foreword to the book in spite of many other demands on his time. To him I owe the quality of life I have today because of his faith in the human brain.

Jennifer Gordon
April 1994

I would like to thank Melita Brown, Head of Speech Pathology at Royal Perth Hospital in Western Australia for her support and encouragement for Speechless to be reprinted.

Thank you to Amie Lees for proof-reading the second edition and being a fun guest. Thank you again to Margaret MacPherson, Dr Rosemary German-Belmont and Yvonne Bryce for their friendship, support and suggestions for the final chapter.

Second Edition
Jennifer Gordon
April 2011

CONTENTS

Foreword by Dr. W. M. Carroll
Preface
Acknowledgements

PRE-STROKE
Chapter One   Fleabites And Sour Wine   1

THE STROKE
Chapter Two   Twenty Questions   12

RECOVERY - THE FIRST SIX MONTHS
Chapter Three   The Birds Are Cawing   25
Chapter Four   Freeway South And Channel Ten   32
Chapter Five   If God Could Hear You Now   41
Chapter Six   Brain Clicks   50
Chapter Seven   Outward Bound   68
Chapter Eight   Ledges   78
Chapter Nine   Rip Van Winkle   88
Chapter Ten   The Mind Boggles   99
Chapter Eleven   Left Luggage   112

RECOVERY AFTER SIX MONTHS
Chapter Twelve   Too Slow   124
Chapter Thirteen   Tin Roofs And Mezzanine Floors   136
Chapter Fourteen   Stretching The Brain   151
Chapter Fifteen   Twenty-Three Years Later   159

Epilogue   164
Further Reading   170

CHAPTER ONE

Fleabites and Sour Wine

At school we used to play a game. If you could die of anything you chose, what would it be? I knew the answer. 'Anything but a stroke'.

At that age, about fourteen I imagined a stroke would turn the hapless victim into a living vegetable utterly dependant on the goodness of others for every requirement – bathing, feeding and dressing.

In 1988, at the age of forty-three, I had a stroke.
In my environment there were quite a few of the conditions that are thought to predispose one to stroke, among them stress and a high-cholesterol diet.

For some people, teaching is not a particularly stressful

occupation. But for me it was. I had taught Science for twelve years at high school, university and a college of advanced education and I believe the stress of those years gradually got the better of me. Certainly, I had not felt constantly tense before I started teaching, when I had worked in a pathology laboratory as a medical scientist.

To give myself a rest from teaching I took a part-time job in the Red Cross Blood Bank. This kind of work should have been a breeze. But my personality had changed. I did not laugh much any more, I was often too tired to sleep and I became intolerant and introverted.

About a year before the stroke a specialist prescribed for me a drug for endometriosis, a gynaecological complaint. I took it for about ten months. This type of drug is known to increase lipids in the blood and an increase in lipids is often associated with an increase in cholesterol. I had never had my cholesterol checked before but it seems I have a genetic predisposition to high cholesterol. It was found to be high after the stroke and I have often wondered if it had been even higher when I was taking the medication.

At the time of my stroke, my exercise programme was poor. I played golf intermittently and I walked – but not very regularly, usually at weekends. I am 160 centimetres tall and my weight (with the aid of the medication I had been taking) had crept up to over 60 kilograms. I did not smoke.

I considered that my diet was adequate although I realise now it was not. I loved full-cream milk, butter, cream and cheese – all the things that contain cholesterol. On the other hand I could easily bypass cakes, soft drinks and fast food. I ate red meat and chicken about six times a week and plenty of vegetables and salads. I did not eat any fish at all, nor did I much care for fruit.

In hindsight the first symptom of my impending stroke occurred at the end of April 1987. I had pins and needles and a feeling of weakness in my right arm. It must have worried me at the time because I wrote in my diary, 'Could it be a symptom of stroke?'.

In mid-1987 I began to think my house was infested with fleas and was convinced my dog and cat were bringing them in. This, in spite of the fact that I could not see any bites. I experienced intense itching, mainly in my legs, face and head. I went to a doctor who gave me an insecticidal cream, with which I practically poisoned myself. I smeared it on my body with careless abandon. The inside of my nose itched very badly and although the cream is not supposed to be used on mucous membranes, I applied it there anyway – to the inside of my nose and to my lips. Fortunately before I could do any more damage I ran out of cream. This terrible itching only occurred when I was in bed and was not there in the morning. I experienced the itching, on and off, right up to the time of the stroke. And then it disappeared.

Meanwhile I rang the local council about the fleas. It did not have a pest controller but sent me what it considered to be the next best thing: a noise abatement officer. There were no fleas to be found.

In December 1987 I began to suffer from a terribly stiff neck. This usually came on while I was lying in bed and I was unable to find a position to ease the discomfort. It felt to me as though my neck and head were slowly silting up: these frightening symptoms and irrational thoughts persisted until the day of the stroke.

From about that time all wine tasted drab and sour. I particularly like red wine but even the best tasted sour. I did not notice it in food, just wine.

Towards the end of 1987 I started looking for another job. My only child Benjamin had gone to England and I missed him very much. I made up my mind to visit him and to do this I needed to be earning more money. I decided to go back to teaching and started at a new school – a private college – in February 1988. This move was to fuel intense worry.

I had a sense of not feeling confident with my preparation for school, a feeling that there was always a bit missing. This led to my staying at home working on my lesson preparation for hours at the weekends as well as during the week. The work became harder and harder to do. It got to the stage where I had to look up course content (which I knew backwards) just before I went into a class. As well as this I had a personality clash with one of my colleagues. This added to the stress of the job.

I began to suffer from sleeplessness. I could not bear the thought of arriving half-asleep for school and having to take classes feeling like a zombie. So I would get off to sleep with the help of a sleeping tablet. I would wake up around one o'clock in the morning with the 'fleabites' driving me crazy to have a glass of (full-cream) milk and another sleeping tablet. It never occurred to me to wonder where the 'bites' had gone in the morning.

I could not relax. Weekends were just days on which I did not have the extra burden of working at the school itself.
With my son away I was alone in the house. I had split up with a man friend of fairly long standing about six months previously. It is said that there is a certain amount of stress attached to living on your own without the benefit of another for a supportive, loving relationship.

There was swelling around my eyes which used to itch and did not look very pleasant. My eyes were particularly swollen at night but I put that down to lack of sleep.

I became very tired but thought it was a symptom of overwork. It would clear up, I felt sure, once I could take a holiday. One day I had arranged to meet my friend Tom after work for drinks and then dinner but I was too tired to go on for dinner. I missed out on all sorts of social activities that way - twilight sailing, dinners and seeing films. I just could not drag myself around.

I slept a great deal. Once while driving back from the country to Perth, I was so overcome with fatigue that I pulled into a truck bay, climbed into the back of my van and slept for an hour. It was only a two hour drive. I had rationalisations for this occasion as I did for everything. It was a hot day and I told myself I had clearly been overdoing it. But I had been quite fresh and rested when I started the journey.

My coordination had suddenly gone haywire about a year before the stroke. I noticed it in my golf swing. It was not just a little bit off, it was right off. There were times when I could not hit the ball at all and I had been playing since I was ten years old. In the twelve months that followed, my game was very haphazard – sometimes fair, sometimes appalling. By June 1988 I could no longer play eighteen holes. I could barely play nine because of the tiredness. Ironically a few weeks before the stroke I had one of my best rounds. It was rather like the true story of a chess-player who checkmated his long-time rival then had a fatal heart attack.

I began to look very unwell. My skin became pasty and my hair impossible: unkempt, no shine and the little muscles that hold the individual hairs up just sagging. I had it cut shorter and shorter and when that did not work I bought a new hairdryer.

Then in May 1988 a large capillary burst in my eye. This frightened me and made me look worse than ever. I was worried enough to see a doctor about that but he assured me it was nothing sinister.

There were nightmares – particularly in the six weeks before the stroke. No sooner had I laid my head down than they would start. Brightly coloured and strangely obscene, in shades of red and purple, they were involved and seemed to last all night. Occasionally, they were quite pleasant but even then they always had an eerie quality. I remember one in which I walked with an unknown lover, around a lake bounded by rhododendrons, in the grounds of a huge mansion made of sandstone. But usually the nightmares were frightening. Sometimes I saw helmeted motorcyclists in military uniform chasing me with sub-machine guns. In one I wandered all night in a vast, empty factory and discovered the body of a murdered man. The dreams were so vivid that I kept on seeing them for seconds after I had woken up.

Once, at the beginning of June, I jumbled the words in a couple of sentences on an overhead transparency I had prepared for my class. I did not realise I had done it at the time but when I spotted it I wondered if my class would notice. They did.

A week or so later, while I was at home preparing another overhead transparency for school my eyes suddenly started troubling me. I could not see the page I was looking at. There was a jagged, green light with fine black edges, outlining a very bright patch of white and vivid pink light in front of my eyes – like the 'balloons' coming out of cartoon characters' mouths only taking up the whole field of view. This was accompanied by an intense feeling of nausea, whereupon I went to bed to lie down.

The room was going round and round as it does when one has a hangover but this was worse – and in any case I had not been drinking. I was very frightened. Again the thought of a stroke crossed my mind. I told myself tremulously it must be migraine but I did not really believe it.

I had only been lying down for a few seconds when the telephone rang. I answered it and it was my friend Rosemary. I opened my mouth to speak - and could not. I managed to make a noise by tapping the receiver against a book to show that I was there at the other end of the telephone. Finally having got my speech back (some ten seconds later) I told her I thought I was having a stroke. I instantly regretted saying it. The thought had just popped out of my mind – where it had lain up to now, stifled and repressed. It certainly had not occurred to me to admit my dark fears to any other person. I quickly tried to cover my tracks – and willed the thought away, like an ostrich with its head in the sand. But I could not stop Rosemary and her husband, Allen, who is a doctor, coming round at once. Allen wanted me to go to hospital but wild horses could not have dragged me away! Had I been in a cooperative frame of mind (I found that the lead-up to the stroke made me very uncooperative) I would probably seen the sense of what they were advising. I reluctantly agreed to go home with them so they could keep their eye on me. They kept telling me I looked unwell but a couple of hot toddies later I felt fine. Allen makes a mean hot toddy.

I experienced occasional losses of speech (about once a week at first) after that incident. I noticed them particularly when I was on the telephone. They became progressively more severe lasting five to ten seconds at a time.

Around this time I also experienced facial twitching. The skin from my nose to my lip would be dragged tight for a few moments, then released.

I would wake in the morning (or in the night) unable to

focus on my digital clock about two metres away. Gradually, after about ten seconds, it would come into clear view. This worried me but the fact that it did eventually come into view seemed to preclude there being anything much physically wrong with my sight.

Since the end of February 1988 I had been suffering from sinusitis accompanied by headaches that became increasingly severe as time went on. I had been to a doctor several times about this. At the end of June I experienced a blinding headache – I literally could not see in front of me when the pain peaked and it was coming in waves. I had to stay in bed for three days. I telephoned my friend Jasmine and asked her if she would come round and make me tea and toast. She did so but she was in a hurry. She had someone sitting in the car ready to go down to Walpole, a town in the South-West of Western Australia. She brought some flowers with her and I said pettishly, 'They give me allergies'. I suppose what I meant was, 'I want you to stay with me and not go rushing off to Walpole'. Jasmine sensibly had telephoned Rosemary and she came round with some other friends of mine, Elizabeth and David. They convinced me I should see a doctor.

It was Sunday and the clinic I normally attended was not staffed at the weekend. We had to ring through to a locum. He established that I was not a child and sounded supremely uninterested in seeing an adult with only a headache. Two hours later he still had not arrived. By that time the headache was beginning to ease. We cancelled the reluctant locum six hours later and I promised my friends that first thing in the morning I would go to my doctor and tell him about my symptoms. I could not squirm out of that one.

I went to the clinic the next morning. Over the previous six months I had been to the doctor nine times mostly because of my headaches which I was convinced were due to sinusitis. As it was such a large practice and because I had to juggle my work commitments to make appointments, I had rarely seen the same doctor twice. But on this occasion my appointment was with the doctor I usually preferred to see.

I complained about the continuous headache, the throbbing in my head and the nausea. In exasperation I flung down on the desk the tablets other doctors had given me - antibiotics for blocked sinuses and analgesics for the headaches. They had not worked at all. The doctor examined my eyes and listened to the carotid artery in my neck. But all my symptoms had gone by then. When he said he thought I had been suffering from a cluster headache I went away thankfully and tried to forget about it.

In retrospect of course I should have taken more notice of my symptoms, especially the neurological ones, and reported these more fully to my doctor. My excuse for inaction was that I was afraid of what the illness might turn out to be. Anyway, I illogically thought, I was too busy to be ill. And it seemed to me the symptoms did not last long enough to be taken seriously.

I now know that these neurological symptoms are called TIA's (transient ischaemic attacks: transient meaning short-term and ischaemic meaning without blood). They are little strokes caused by a momentary blockage to an artery in the brain. Sometimes these blockages are due to small fragments of fatty tissue or blood clots, called emboli, that have broken off a hardening artery. They are swept along by the blood until subsequent divisions of the arteries become too narrow and a blockage occurs.

TIA's are a warning that should be heeded, for if left unattended they may lead to a stroke.

The neurological symptoms I experienced were:
- pins and needles and weakness in my arm;
- excruciating headache;
- disturbances of vision that cleared within a few minutes: 'balloons' or flashes of light in the eyes and inability to focus;
- nausea and dizziness;
- the feeling that the room was spinning;
- lack of coordination;
- speech loss;
- changes in the taste of things (like wine);
- poor decision-making ability;
- facial twitches.

Taken all together my symptoms presented a formidable group – so much so that I wonder how I could have missed them. I had taught Human Biology after all. Of the other symptoms I experienced, some may have had nothing to do with the stroke.

Some people project a positive image that may mislead a busy doctor. I am one of them. If I could have put my fear to one side and any unconscious mental blocks I might have had I would have been better able to explain my symptoms – at least in the early part of the illness. But with the ultimate failure in my decision-making ability I was unable to see things in a realistic light. I had had to be told by my friends to see a doctor and I had only done so to keep them happy and to stop them nagging me.

My friend Yvonne later said my personality changed during the months leading up to the stroke. I became moody and withdrawn, easily upset with people. Alan, another friend said he thought I had gone mad because I was so obsessive about the person at school with whom I was having a personality clash. That situation certainly added to my stress but I believe it just brought on the inevitable a little sooner. Rosemary and Allen noticed a change in me as well. So did other friends but they were too polite to say so.

Shortly after that visit to the doctor, three of us – Rosemary, another friend Phil and I – mounted an expedition to Rottnest, a little island due west of Perth and about half an hour by hydrofoil. It is lovely there in the winter when it is not crowded.

On Rottnest I was constantly troubled by loss of speech. It had accelerated from approximately once a week to four or five times in an hour while I tried to make conversation with people around me. Phil was worried about me, she said what was happening to my speech was not normal.

In the lounge of the hotel that night, sitting around an open fire, I almost felt back to normal but it was short-lived. I had a nightmare that night and spent the next day feeling haunted and withdrawn. Luckily I got back to Perth without mishap. If my stroke had occurred on Rottnest Island it would have been far more problematic.

At the beginning of July I began to become confused about whether to stop at traffic lights or not. Did green mean I was to stop? Or was it red? I had to pull up at traffic lights with a skid several times on my way to the city-suburb of Fremantle about three days before the stroke.

Hiraeth, my Siamese cat became very concerned about me. He followed me about and slept on my bed and as he is not normally a very demonstrative cat I was pleased. A day or so before the stroke I was so tired that I decided to take a quick sleep before I fed Hiraeth and my corgi dog, Maggie. That thought was scarcely in my mind when Maggie started to whimper strangely and Hiraeth began to yowl. Possibly they saw something distorted in my expression. I had never heard them do that before and they never did it again.

CHAPTER TWO

Twenty Questions

On 6th July 1988, it happened. Rosemary had come round and we went for a walk. We then made a cup of tea and I was still sitting in my chair. I felt nothing, no sudden squeeze or pain in my brain, nothing to mark the terrible thing that happened next.

My whole right arm, without my volition, raised itself off my lap and twisted backwards and forwards and sideways. It was as if I were a cow that had just been slaughtered. I have seen slaughterers put a wire in the hole caused by the 'captive bolt' in the cow's head and twist it around. First one leg shoots out, then another. That is what my arm felt like, as if somebody else was moving the wire. At the same time my fingers flexed and pointed and my palm writhed around first to face me, then away. I watched it all in fascination.

After a few minutes the arm settled down to a steady trembling. I was not aware of the trembling at the time nor of my mouth which drooped on the right. I staggered when I tried to walk on my now enfeebled right leg.

From then on speech was completely lost. I became curiously docile. Rosemary took charge straight away and fortunately she did not panic.

It was quite a cold day and Rosemary tried to slip a cardigan over my shoulders. No matter how hard she tried she could not get it to stay on; my shoulders were lifeless. I looked at them in curious fascination as if they too did not belong to me. Rosemary solved the problem by helping me to the car, settling me in the passenger seat and arranging the cardigan around me.

She asked me where my doctor had his rooms. I think I just looked pleasantly interested. She tried another tack, 'Which way do we go?' I said nothing. 'Left or right?' she tried. My gestures meant very little and I indicated right or left with little regard for accuracy. Consequently Rosemary initially went round in circles. At this juncture let it be said that Rosemary has a terrible sense of direction herself but even she realised something was wrong when we passed my house for the third time. I could picture the route we should have taken but telling someone else was another story. Rosemary then looked up the address in the telephone book. When we pulled up at the traffic lights outside the surgery, I was well aware of where we were but I let Rosemary keep on driving. I could not think of any way of telling her we were there. Rosemary,thank goodness is intuitive. Once past the traffic lights she stopped. I must have nodded my head when she asked, 'Was it over there?'.

We came to realise later that I would nod and shake my head indiscriminately whatever the question.

We eventually saw my doctor and he wrote me a letter of referral to a Perth hospital the Queen Elizabeth 11 Medical Centre (QE11). We arrived at QE11 at 2-00 pm and Rosemary did not leave until midnight. I was quite convinced it was all a big mistake and that they were making a big fuss over nothing. I wanted to go home.

The specialist neurologist, Dr B, swept in accompanied by two residents. I knew as soon as I saw him that I would like and trust him. Thoughts of leaving the hospital quickly vanished and all I wanted to do was get well again. I was in a much more settled frame of mind now. Dr B talked to me directly even though I could not talk back. I cannot overemphasise what a difference that made. Even though I could not speak, Dr B was taking me seriously. I still felt just the same inside. I could understand what people were saying to me; I just could not communicate with them.

Shortly after that I went to X-ray on a stretcher. A white-coated woman appeared at the door wheeled me in and told me to get off the bed 'to the right hand side'. I noted the instruction and promptly got off to the left. This in fact was fairly difficult because they had pulled the stretcher up close to the left-hand wall. Not wishing to appear foolish, I clawed at the wall and succeeded eventually in moving the bed just enough so that I could lever myself out. The woman and her colleagues pushed the bed back saying, 'No! we said right'. I thought a little wondering where I had gone wrong and tried again. I did the same thing. This time they let me clamber round the bed and feeling very pleased with myself I made my way to the place where they wanted me to stand. There was no mistake about that because one of the radiographers was standing there already.

An orderly took me up to the ward and I was given a private room on the seventh floor with a truly magnificent view of the Swan River, which flows through Perth.

A nursing sister called Julie took my blood pressure and pulse, looked at the pupils of my eyes, checked my grip and tested how hard I could push with my feet, first the left foot (the undamaged one) and then the right. I could not tell that there was any difference between my two sides even much later. This was what they were looking for. I started to recover from the paralysis in my right arm and leg within ten hours (I was told). Apparently if the paralysis goes quickly one has a good chance of recovering full use of the limbs. But Phil told me my right hand was still quivering when she came to see me the next day.

Dr B came in and spoke kindly to me. He explained about the heparin drip that they were about to put into my arm. This was to make my blood less able to clot – 'thinner'. I was glad of that kindness. A Jewish doctor wearing an embroidered skull cap and one of those who had examined me in Casualty easily put the cannula into my arm. I stress 'easily' because I would not have known just how difficult the procedure was had I not had three doctors after that who could not get the drip in at all. (A ferocious woman doctor got it in in the end.)

I was told afterwards that I would not turn my head to the right and I ignored anyone standing on my right. This lasted a few days. When Rosemary stood on my right side and spoke to me I acted as if she were not there. Julie, at the foot of the bed, suggested Rosemary should stand on my left. I noticed her at once then. Apparently this is a common thing in people with paralysis on one side. Anything happening on the damaged side is ignored.

I was sent for a CAT-scan – whereupon inexplicably I started to sob. I could not stop myself; it was terribly embarrassing. I came to associate being over-emotional and sobbing with anything new I was asked to do. Down I went, sobbing, to the scanning unit located on the first floor. People must have thought that I was upset or frightened by the thought of a scan. But I did not feel particularly upset.

The most likely thing (I was told) that would have caused me to have had a stroke was a clot lodged in the brain. The scan was to discover whether there were any more clots lurking in my body.

I was parked in a waiting room next to the scanning unit. When it was time for my scan I was transferred to a smaller bed that slides into the large tube structure where the scanning is done. The soft lighting had a calming effect. I was left on my own in the room. Everyone went out and I heard a disembodied voice telling me what the operators were doing.

The whole procedure took about twenty minutes. I am a nervous sort of person so I kept my eyes tightly shut.

CAT stands for 'computer assisted tomography'. A series of X-ray pictures is taken in slices very close together so that there is a complete picture of, for example, the inside of my head. In my case the doctors were following the internal carotid artery from the neck to where it had become blocked by a clot deep inside my brain.

My world was full of shadows. I was experiencing tunnel vision. For a time it was as if the whole room was covered in the shadows from a soft bedside lamp.

The next day I had a bee in my bonnet. I thought I knew exactly what was wrong with me, if only I could tell them!

Two years before I had inadvertently left a tampon in place for four weeks and had developed toxic shock syndrome. At that time I had a sinus-like headache and fever and I felt weak and dizzy with foul material running down the back of my throat. It cleared up when I took antibiotics then returned again when I stopped taking them. The symptoms went at once when the tampon was removed.

I had a period at the time of the stroke. I was convinced the same thing had happened and that I was suffering from toxic shock syndrome again. But I could not make anyone listen to me because I could not speak. I had never felt so helpless in my life. I was unable to move and powerless to communicate. I lay there believing I knew what was the cause of the trouble and watching them as they were misled into thinking a dozen things that the illness was not (according to me). I managed to convey to Rosemary - possibly by means of anguished facial expressions and a few tears - that I thought the 'stroke' was something entirely different. She wrote it down for me. She was endlessly patient with her 'twenty questions' approach.

Rosemary: Are you worried about the stroke?
Jenny: [Flinging arms about.]
Rosemary: Something else?
Jenny: [Grovel, grovel.]
Rosemary: Something that's happened recently?
Jenny: [Manic smile.]
Rosemary: Five years ago?
Jenny: [Confusion – I recognised the word 'year' but I didn't like five of them.]

She put a written version of our 'conversation' in the nurses' station to await Dr B. when he next came onto the ward. I was disappointed when I saw what she had written. Only two sentences. Funny: I thought I told her more than that.

The Jewish doctor came in then and I thought, 'Now's my chance'. I beckoned the poor unsuspecting fellow over to the side of my bed threw back the covers and pointed to my pelvis. He drew back in horror – and declined! I was very embarrassed. Nothing daunted I waited till all was quiet that night and then set to work to get the tampon out. (It did not occur to me that the tampon I was wearing because of my period would not have been the one causing the 'toxic shock syndrome'). It was exceedingly difficult to say the least, with my maimed hand but I persevered. I could not make my right hand do what I wanted it to do at all. I don't know how long it took me to do it but I got it out at last. Eureka! I grabbed the tampon firmly in both hands and rang for the night nurse. She came fussing in with her torch and beheld me grinning wildly from all my exertions. I unclasped my hands at the crucial moment and thrust the tampon at her. She screamed. Much put out I put it in the drawer of the unit beside me and went to sleep.

Shortly after that Rosemary's husband, Allen, came to see me. He was very concerned. I threw my arms around him and burst into tears as usual. When my tears had subsided to a sniff he brought out a notebook and wrote the alphabet in capital letters. I was delighted and pounced on the notebook eager to make up for lost time. I pointed to the letters then started again, and again. No good: it was not going to be that easy. I could picture what I wanted to say to some extent but I could not get it to the outside. The letters of the alphabet did not help at all.

The shadows were very intense that day. I could not see the door and I did not recognise the bedside table. Somehow I seemed much nearer to the end of the bed than I had before. In fact things were thoroughly distorted.

People said to me later that it must have been very frustrating for me to have been like that but in a way it was not. I was in such a desperate plight that I had very little time to

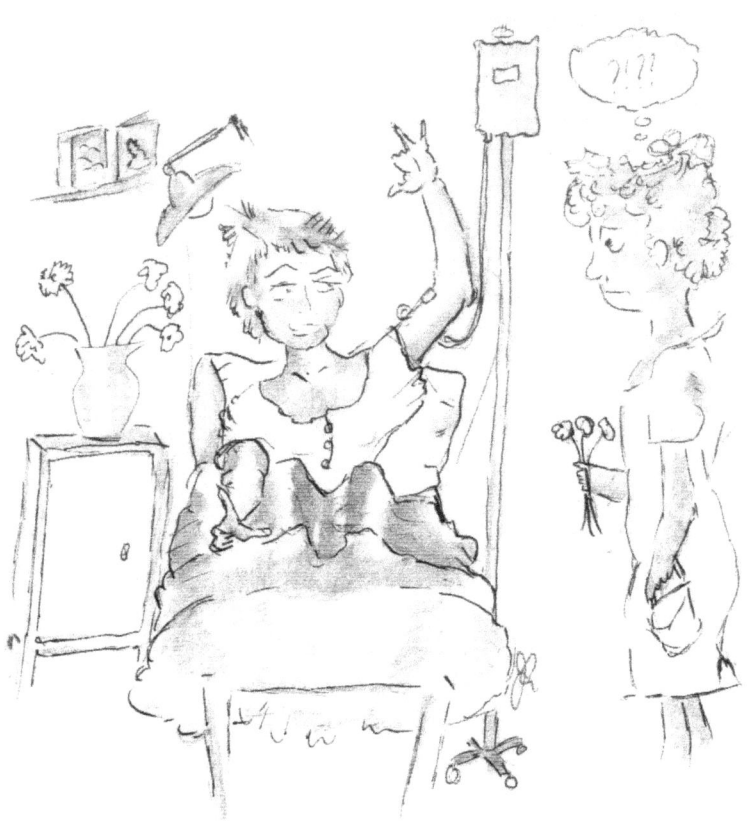

'Meaningless gestures'

think about it. My frustration was to come much later.

On the third day in hospital I was sent for another CAT-scan and the orderly again wheeled me down on my bed.

Then graduating to a wheelchair another orderly took me for an EEG (electroencephalogram) which involved placing sticky jelly on my head and attaching electrodes to it. This procedure did not hurt. Neither did the lights they shone at me at different frequencies. But what did hurt was the way the orderly carelessly pushed me back to the ward. Laughing and joking with his cronies in the lift, he steered me into the sliding door. We skidded up the corridor to my room nearly missed it and 'wham' into the door jamb we went. Later I thought that I would not have minded so much if he had even acknowledged me and said, 'Hello' when he first started pushing but he did not.

I was very accepting of all the things they did. I was too confused to be otherwise.

When all the tests were finished the woman doctor told me, 'You have had a stroke'. I was furious. I cried bitter tears of disbelief because I still thought I knew what was really wrong with me. It was toxic shock syndrome of course!

But when Dr B. came to see me I finally believed him and he explained how it had happened. A blood clot from another part of my body that had formed a fatty plaque had become detached and had lodged in the left-hand side of my brain thus blocking the middle cerebral artery. The left-hand side of the brain controls the right side of the body and the major speech centres. So I had lost the use of my right side (arm, leg and face) as well as my speech.

Dr B. said the clot would not move and I would not have any further trouble from it. It was only if another clot formed in another part of my body, that there would be a problem. He was very convincing. My toxic shock hypothesis was fading fast. The Jewish doctor must have overcome his horror enough to understand my concerns and pass them on to his superior. Dr B. ordered an X-ray to be taken of my pelvic region. Even though I knew by then I was probably wrong I was very happy that he was listening to me even in my confused state. My first reactions to him in Casualty were confirmed and I knew that here indeed was a man I liked and trusted. It was a tremendous load off my mind and I settled down to the job of getting well.

But soon I began to get really depressed. A speech pathologist called to see me and I scowled and refused to cooperate. She obviously had better things to do than spend time with such a blatantly ungrateful patient and she went quietly away. And I went back to my blues. As Shakespeare said, 'And with old woes new waile my deare times waste...'. I wallowed in my misery. I was even unable to pray. That struck me as odd but as praying is thinking in words it was not surprising. 'Well, God will have to do without prayers', I decided ungraciously.

I was lying there thinking murderous thoughts. 'What's the good of life if you can't speak, you can't think and your arm and leg don't work? As soon as I can get to the window I will throw myself out of it', I promised. I remembered a book I had read recently about a woman who had paraplegia (from an accident). She allowed herself one day to wallow in the feeling of loss and hopelessness and then would not entertain such thoughts again. It seemed a jolly good idea to me, especially the first part. So I let myself go and cried all day.

Later a ward assistant said to me in disapproving tones, 'You really dropped your bundle, didn't you?'. All I could do was glare at her thinking, 'if only I could give you a piece of my mind, you rancid little woman'. I did not seem to be able to get along with either the ward assistants or the kitchen assistants.

Elizabeth and Rosemary put a notice on my door: 'Mrs Gordon would like tea with milk and no sugar, please'. Some of the kitchen assistants still left me the wrong thing and some of them stared wonderingly at the notice and did not come in at all. So I limped to the door removed the notice and took my chances.

During the first few days I went to sleep with the aid of what I thought was a sleeping capsule. It certainly had that effect on me. A sister broke the capsule which I then held under my tongue. The next thing I knew it was morning. I found out later that this drug was 'Adalat' a vasodilator and calcium channel inhibitor that minimised the effect of the stroke.

On the fourth night after the stroke I had a 'mind picture'. These are dreams but mind pictures are more real to me than dreams are. They make more of an impression and one wakes up thinking about them. That is how I distinguished between mind pictures and dreams. In this mind picture I was in a room with six or seven other people whom I could see clearly. They were people I did not know but it was a pleasant enough scene. And in it I was talking again, not perfectly, but talking nevertheless. I woke up that morning with a great sense of peace. I did not worry after that, I just let time flow on past.

Elizabeth often came to see me at lunchtime as she worked in research at QE11. She said, 'You will get your speech back, you know'. It was the first time I had heard that I might or maybe the first time I had *listened* when it was said. One does not tend to dwell on the outcomes of stroke before it happens to one and although I had dealt with stroke when I was teaching Human Biology it had not been in much detail. I thought the damage done by the stroke would be with me forever. Elizabeth's words were a revelation.

Elizabeth brought me a tape recorder and some tapes and I

learned two things. The first was that I could no longer work a simple instrument. I had to ask somebody to turn the volume down because I could not do it myself. There were three small knobs on the top of the machine but I could not fathom them out.

The second thing I learned was that I did not enjoy music any more. In fact I was not to recover my feeling for music until about two years after the stroke. I could listen to music bar by bar – I was not tone deaf – but each bar was totally unrelated to the one before it and the one after it. It did nothing for me emotionally. I could play my Welsh choirs, or the Mendelssohn violin concerto or Rod Stewart without being moved.

One of the night sisters gave me a great deal of encouragement. Her name was Hannah. She talked to me at a normal pace and asked, 'Why aren't you seeing a speech pathologist?'. There was no need to talk slower and louder than usual to me as some people did. I could hear well enough and I could process what I was hearing. I just could not speak or communicate myself. I acted as dumbly as I could for once glad that I could not say anything. I would not have wanted to tell Hannah I had behaved so badly when the speech pathologist came that she had left. Hannah reported her opinion that I needed speech therapy with the result that the speech pathologist visited me again. It was five days after the stroke and I was glad of her this time.

I soon noticed the television up above my bed. It had all the usual channels and a special hospital channel. I never tired of the movie *Local Hero*. And some part of my brain understood and enjoyed the hospital programmes on 'Diabetic Food' and 'Heart Disease'.

My cholesterol level was 7.3 millimoles per litre (the recommended level was 4.5 millimoles per litre at the time) so the dietician came to see me and I was put on a low-cholesterol diet. And it seemed I would have to stay on it. At that time I was not eating much at all. The food was quite good at QE11 but when everyone else was enjoying fish and chips I had to have steamed fish and no chips. I lost weight.

Six days after the stroke I was allowed out of bed to stumble round my room. I was trying to apply mascara with my left hand when my friend Duncan came to see me. I had not seen him for over six months and I was very pleased. So what did I do? I sobbed. 'When you are ready to come out of hospital' he said 'you can come and stay with me'. It was a wonderful offer from a true friend. By the time I came out of hospital however I was able to live on my own again.

At the time of Duncan's visit I had a slightly curling lip, a noticeable limp and still very little control over my shaking hand. I had not spoken for six days: I could not even grunt. Elizabeth had brought me some makeup, a photo of my son and clothes from home. I smudged the lipstick on the right-hand side of my mouth but not on the left. I did not notice the smudge. I bought a nail file, a razor and a pair of scissors from the volunteer trolley. With careless abandon I shaved my legs and (I had slight movement in my right hand) cut my nails. A few days later what had appeared to me to be a perfect job seemed suddenly ragged. The nails were very uneven – even though I had taken great care over them. As for the shaving I had taken even more care with that, but there were little scratches and gouges all over my legs.

Suddenly I was able to make a noise! It was only a sort of 'Agghhing' noise but I was well on my way to speech again. The speech pathologist came that afternoon on the twelfth of July and I was able to dazzle her with my 'Agghh'.

CHAPTER THREE

The Birds are Cawing

Shauna, my first speech pathologist told me I was suffering from speech dyspraxia and aphasia. She was highly organised. She began by bringing me an exercise book with the main points about dyspraxia glued to the front cover. I could show this to friends who came to visit me.

It said:

In this disorder the patient has difficulty in voluntarily producing speech sounds. Sometimes a sound or a word may be said easily and correctly and at other times it may not. The way the sounds and words are said can vary greatly. A patient may sound very hesitant while he is groping to make the right sounds. In Speech Dyspraxia the muscles are not weak or paralysed but they are not under the control of the speaker. Aphasia is a disruption of communication, which may include many skills, such as not understanding what people say, and not expressing oneself through speech or gesture, reading, writing and calculation.

I struggled with 'fall' and 'fish' and 'fine feathers' till I was exhausted with the effort. But if I thought that was hard just wait till I got to 'visit Vera' and 'vote for value'. Shauna helped by making faces of the sounds for me to copy.

At this time I began to write with my left hand. Rosemary got me a card to write to Ben. She left saying, 'You have a think about what you want to put in it'. I thought and thought. The trouble was that the thoughts kept evaporating when I tried to get them into more concrete forms.

I could imagine a place in my brain where my imaginings and thoughts formed; another where they were assembled into readable order; and one in which they were delivered as speech, writing or thinking. It was between the first two – between the 'thoughts forming' and the 'assembly into order' – where my trouble lay.

So needless to say I had not got anything down on paper by the time my friend arrived the next day. I was still puzzling over it and thinking, 'Any time now and I'll get it'.

I had been in hospital for several days by this time and I still had not notified the school that I was not coming back; I had been so sure I would be up and around in a few days. But my will began to weaken. Rosemary urged me to let her tell them so that they could get a replacement. I eventually agreed. The doctors showed every indication of keeping me in hospital for the foreseeable future.

Upon being told of my illness colleagues from the school came to see me. Waving my arms about I tried to assure them it was only a temporary lapse: I would be back at school in no time. But still I had no speech.

Rosemary telephoned England where Ben was staying with my mother. Naturally they were both distressed to hear what had happened and Ben wanted to come back to Perth. I managed to convey to Rosemary that I did not want him to come. There was nothing he could do to help and from now on I could be expected to get better. He was in the middle of intensive training, hoping to join the Royal Marines. Through Rosemary I assured him that my friends were taking good care of me.

For the first two weeks in hospital I seemed to spend most of my time working out how to shower myself and wash my hair with my fuddled brain and my left hand. At first a nurse went with me to the shower and I had to sit down. I found this demeaning but the nurse was very encouraging and said I would be standing in no time – and I was. The next day I was a bit wobbly but undoubtedly standing. I am still at a loss to explain how I got my nightdress on over my heparin drip. By the time the drip was taken out I still was not very intelligent about things so I never did find out.

The heparin drip was worked by mains electricity and had a short-term battery backup. I would unplug the drip stand when I wanted to go to the toilet or to take a shower and then forget to plug it back in. The battery would get low and the unit would respond with a nervous, high-pitched buzz. They kept telling me to plug it back in. One day it finally made sense – I remembered to plug it back in all by myself. I remember the sense of achievement.

I drew pictures for Dr B. He would draw a clock with hands on it or house shapes. I had to draw the same thing. For some reason I found it easier to draw my copy directly beneath the doctor's prototype rather than alongside it. This was another neurological test to see if I was acknowledging my right side. If I were not the houses and clocks would not be completed.

About two weeks after the stroke I was moved out of my private room and into a ward with four people. I was beginning to feel a lot better – the headaches, nausea, stiff neck and spinning sensations had all disappeared entirely when I had the stroke – I felt ready for some company so I was pleased with the move. That evening three of us set off around the wards to the flower room with me dragging the drip behind me. We only walked four sides of two wards but it was enough to tire me out and make me glad to get back to bed. Up to then I had only tried walking to the nurses' station desk and back to my room, a matter of twenty feet.

My friend, Alan was surprised when he saw me. He said, 'The worried look is all gone from your face'; it was replaced he said, by 'euphoria'. I can only think that the damage affecting my speech had also isolated the fore-brain; and with it the forebrain's guilts and inhibitions. Exaggeration apart I was certainly not unhappy. The last time Alan had been with me I was obsessive and worried about the person at school who I thought was trying to discredit me.

Shauna brought a new toy for my speech pathology session: a tape recorder that played one or two words. It was wonderfully simple to use (I was still uneasy with complicated machinery). You fed in a big card with the word on it. The machine then said the word twice leaving time for you to mumble your own version in between. Shauna had written 'HELLO', 'GOODBYE', 'I'M TIRED' and 'JENNIFER' on the cards. I had great difficulty at first but Shauna left the machine with me over the weekend by the end of which I could say them all – even the hardest, 'JENNIFER'.

I began to feel as though when I woke up each morning I had got over a new hurdle in my speech. Every day it got better. I looked forward to Shauna's visits. She came every day to see me and there was often homework to do. I got four out of ten for the first lot of word-finding exercises I did. I had to match 'millionaire' with something applicable. All the words looked to me as if they could match. I could read them; it was just that they did not mean anything to me in terms of 'rightness'. I eventually picked 'expensive' for 'millionaire'. What did I choose for 'rich'? That's easy: 'cake'.

About three weeks after the stroke I wrote my first letter to Ben and my mother. It was a joint letter as I found it was too tiring to write individual letters. I do not remember writing very much – just a line – but I addressed it myself and remembered the stamp. A little while later I wrote to my friend Tom as well. Tom had been to Europe and did not know I was ill. The letter read: 'I have been ill but I'm all right now.' I can just imagine him receiving that letter with the shaky, unformed handwriting and the cryptic message. I would have preferred it, if I had been Tom, not to have received such a letter at all!

Three students from my school sent me a lovely bouquet of roses and carnations. I could not look at them without a lump coming to my throat and they lasted for ages. I set about writing a thank you note. All the ward helped me because I could not think of any words to describe the flowers. Mary, a fellow patient, offered 'beautiful' and someone else suggested 'gorgeous'. If I could retrieve the word in the first place provided it was not too long I would be able to spell it. I sent the letter off with a considerable glow of satisfaction.

Meanwhile in speech pathology, I had progressed to sentence completion. This was very difficult. 'The birds are

_____'. I almost wore out my meagre supplies of energy and concentration over this one. 'The birds are cawing', I wrote triumphantly. Satisfied that I had done the right thing with that one, I went on. 'The wind is _____.' But I could not get 'cawing' out of my mind. By dint of concentration I dragged my mind away and settled on: 'The wind is breezy'. Shauna said that was not correct but she was very tactful about it.

I just could not handle figures. Shauna showed me a simple equation like 2,086 subtract 1,086. I looked at it in puzzlement. I tried adding it and arrived at a total of 106. She tried again with simpler figures. I had no idea whether I was dividing, multiplying, subtracting or adding. But I had confidence that the figure I arrived at was the right one. It was in this spirit that I gave Rosemary the card to my bank account and my PIN number. Poor Rosemary – after three tries the automatic teller gobbled up the card. Of course I had given her the wrong number.

Elizabeth had taken Maggie home to her place and was looking after her. She told me that as soon as her friend's daughter, Michelle, came back from holiday she would move into my house and look after Maggie and Hiraeth. I was beside myself with worry about Hiraeth. It was two weeks now since the stroke. It was winter and he could not get into the house because there was no cat door. He had not had his vaccinations for the things that cat-flesh is heir to. I did not know if he was being fed.

Eventually I prevailed on Rosemary to take my worries seriously. I should point out that Rosemary hates and fears cats; she has a phobia about them and she cannot believe that anyone can actually like them. I drew a cat in my notebook to emphasise what I could not tell her in my practically non-existent speech. She shuddered and promptly forgot my request in her efforts to erase the memory of my cat picture. It was as though I had just asked an arachnophobe to take care of my bird-eating spider. I need not have worried about Hiraeth. Terry, my neighbour was looking after my house and his son Jason was feeding Hiraeth. Also Jasmine had taken Hiraeth to the vet and organised his injections. They did a good job, Hiraeth was fat and well.

Two and a half weeks after the stroke the heparin drip was removed from my arm and I was allowed out of hospital for the weekend. I was staying with Rosemary and Allen on the day that Michelle moved into my house. Michelle was a veterinary student so I felt that the animals were in good hands. At last things at home seemed to be coming together.

CHAPTER FOUR

Freeway South and Channel Ten

The angiogram was to be an unspeakably awful part of my treatment. The registrar came to tell me about it three weeks after my stroke. The procedure was voluntary but they recommended it because it would confirm their diagnosis of what had caused the stroke. 'If it was a blood clot', the registrar said, 'that had lodged and become settled, it would be the best prognosis for you'. That way they would know (provided another blood clot from some other part of the body did not get lodged in the brain) that I was cured.

I had a day to think about it then the registrar came back with a consent form for me to sign. He had already outlined the risk I would be taking: that if the clot had not settled I might have another stroke. 'But you are in the best place if that remote possibility happened, aren't you?', he said.

Dr B. explained it all to me again when he came in later. There was no possibility that I did not fully understand what was going to happen to me. And I could have said, 'No'. It would have been easy to have taken advantage of a patient whose command of English was zero but whose thinking remained nearly unimpaired on some levels. It was to those 'thinking levels' that Dr B spoke.

I was under the impression that Dr B said I was to have a sedative straight away to relax me for the procedure. But an hour went past then another and they still did not come. My poor, addled brain thrashed about and I became more nervous by the minute. Why didn't I tell somebody? Well, I just did not think of it. That was one of the hard things I had to come to terms with, I simply did not think of obvious things.

Eventually the nurses thought of it themselves but by that time I was so distraught and willing it to work so quickly that it did not seem to be working at all. I wanted to get off the bed and go home. The sister in the angiogram room tut-tutted because the required shaving had not been done up on the ward and I was not properly 'prepared' – like some oven-ready chicken. I was convinced that I would never see my son again and naturally I sobbed over this. As they carried me into the angiogram theatre the sedative began to work at last.

In fact it worked so well that I managed to get thoroughly confused over what was happening. I understood that they were putting a cannula into the right femoral artery (in the groin). But after that, my reasoning got very hazy. I imagined that the femoral artery led straight to the heart. This was incorrect and had I been less groggy from the sedative and from the stroke itself I would have known it. The femoral artery is the one leading from the heart feeding the right leg with fresh blood. In the angiogram procedure the heart is bypassed via another artery then the cannula is led into the internal carotid artery, which in turn leads into the brain.

But I was waiting for the cannula to pierce my heart and I imagined it slowly winding its inexorable way through my body. I did not watch the television monitor I found that I had lost interest in everything except trying to survive.

There were two doctors talking in low tones. I could not hear what they were saying. I conceived the idea that the one who had 'my life in his hands' was a learner and I tried to protest but a sister stepped in and tried to calm me down. By this time the wire had acquired the dimensions of a werewolf's stake about to pierce my heart. I shut my eyes and waited for them to realise that they were going the wrong way. By that time it would be too late for me.

Then all of a sudden they reached the part where the artery enters the skull and they told me to cough to help get the cannula through more easily. I was a bit puzzled, I wondered how they had got past my heart but felt dizzy with relief that I had made it. If I had stopped to think I might have been more worried that they were messing about in my brain. Fortunately that thought did not occur to me.

After it was all over I had an attack of palpitations. That was the last straw. Never having had palpitations before I thought I was dying.

I was wheeled out into another room where Julie, my favourite ward sister, was waiting to collect me. I was in delayed shock. I could not be comforted and cried as though my heart would break. Julie looked enquiringly at the other sister, who said, 'I don't know what upset her, she was all right in there'.

Once I had got over the experience of the angiogram, I started to read a book. I bought myself a Mills and Boon novel *Cage of Ice* from the volunteer trolley. My eyes were blurred from the stroke. If I closed one eye and then the other I could tell the blurring was worse on the right side than on the left. But the left one was fairly bad at that stage too. I had had good eyesight before the stroke and had not needed to wear glasses. I found that after the stroke I could see the page quite well if I held the book further away than usual. But that was not the only problem. Not being able to concentrate was another. I could only read a paragraph then I would collapse from sheer exhaustion and sleep for a while. However, Shauna encouraged me to read and I managed to wander through *Cage of Ice* – missing pages and whole chapters here and there – by the time I left QE11. I was glad of the Mills and Boon predictability knowing that if I missed part of the plot it could easily be picked up further along. It was very restful reading – if you can describe reading a sentence or two and then sleeping as 'restful reading'. I was later able to recall the main gist of the plot even though I had been unable to follow the story at the time.

One day a few weeks after I had been in hospital, Elizabeth and a friend of hers came to see me. They were talking about a shoe sale and trying to remember a particular brand of shoe they had seen. Without thinking about it I said, 'Jane Debster' and it happened to be right! Elizabeth looked at me in astonishment – I had not said anything clever since I had been in hospital – and she commented, 'Out of the mouths of babes and sucklings...'. That incident was very important to me because I was absolutely certain that I had not picked the

RECOVERY - THE FIRST SIX MONTHS

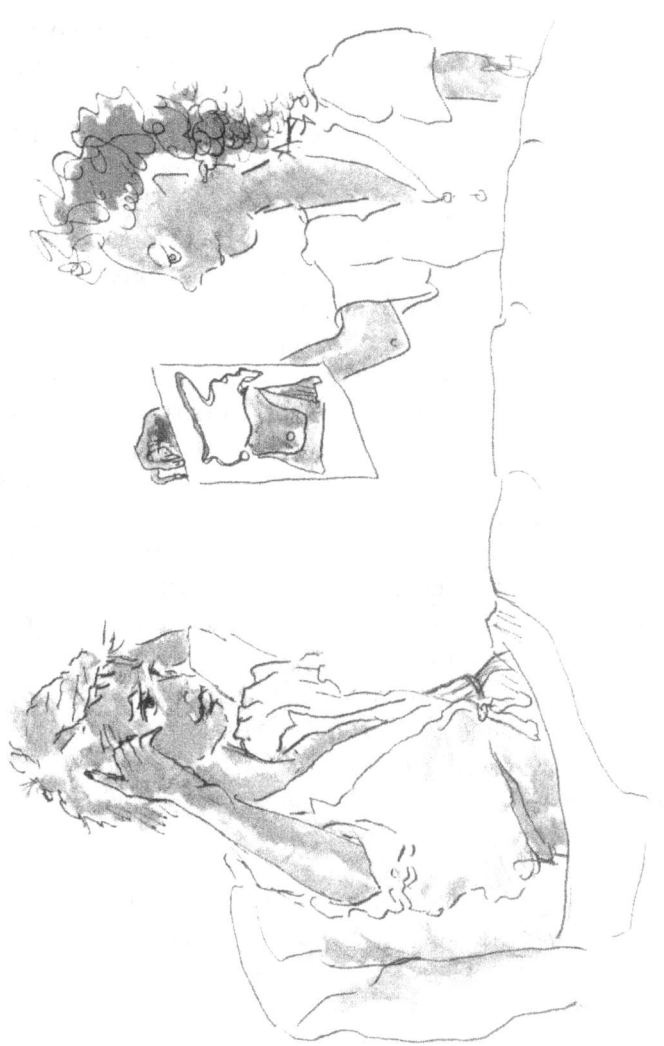

'Don't tell me… it's used for… it's a …'

word up from the television or from people talking around me. It must have come to me from somewhere within my own brain. I had a feeling that I knew a lot of words somewhere in my brain if only I could get at them. It was really an uncanny feeling. I could sometimes say if the word I was looking for began with a C or an S and I could even tell how long the word was. Everyone has those sorts of experiences – but not for ordinary words like 'chair' or 'sink'. The next day I was idly picturing a place at which I used to work giving myself a mind's-eye tour round the familiar laboratories and I said to myself quite distinctly, 'scintillation counter'! And I know that I had not picked up that from television. (A scintillation counter is a piece of laboratory equipment that used to be used for measuring radioactively-labelled materials such carbon, C-14, in fluids, such as serum.)

Shauna and I had moved on in speech therapy. I cannot emphasise enough how important the speech pathologists were in my recovery – first Shauna and later Kathryn, Chris, Suzanne, Isobel, Jan and Melita. Just when I was feeling stuck in some groove they would think of something else to try with me. I found their sessions exhausting.

Shauna showed me a picture of a handbag. I knew what it was. It was stored in my memory – somewhere. Shauna taught me to 'gesture' it first of all. Could I gesture it? I sat glumly looking at it, trying oh so hard to think what one does with a handbag. Shauna 'gestured' it herself, in mime, putting the strap on her shoulder and patting the bag where it lay invisibly against her hip. Of course why had I not thought of that? Then she asked me to 'describe' it. Again nothing. I waved my arms around a good deal in imitation of her gesture but that was all. I had to be prompted. Shauna suggested, 'Say what it can be "used for" and what it is "made of"'.

We only had time to get through the handbag and a picture of an apple before it was time for Shauna to go. I could not describe the apple either [it was red and shiny] much less tell her what it was used for. The next day however, I could do the exercise quite well.

It seemed that I had to keep on exhausting myself otherwise my brain would 'sleep' and I would find it more difficult to 'awaken' it again. It seemed to be a continual process of exercise then sleep. Much like any other organ of the body being trained my brain gradually became more and more fit.

Four weeks after the stroke Duncan took me shopping. I wanted to buy a nightdress and some vitamin C. It was winter, a lot of people had colds and influenza and I did not want that on top of everything else. The shopping centre was busy because it was Saturday and lunchtime. I exhausted myself over choosing the nightdress. The stroke had knocked out my decision-making abilities and I could not make up my mind which nightdress to buy. I could have chosen anything and it would have done the job for my stay in hospital. Duncan was really very good. He hovered in kitchenware and only looked at his watch twice.

At the checkout I fumbled and dropped my purse. I was looking for my credit card and with a shaking hand presented it to the girl. She looked suspiciously at me but did not say anything. I managed to sign it with a trembling hand but it did not go through to the copies underneath, so I had to go through the whole embarrassing procedure again. The girl looked at the signature, looked at my red face and looked at Duncan – and decided to let it pass. Duncan looks the picture of respectability. While I was waiting for him to come out of the greengrocery section I with my tunnel vision idly pushed the trolley into the oncoming stream of shopper traffic and stopped them dead. I did not see them until it was too late. The buzz of angry shoppers hit me. I panicked and did not know what to do about it. Fortunately Duncan smiling apologetically rescued me.

I was particularly upset by the shop assistant's reaction in the pharmacy where I went to buy the vitamin C. Admittedly I made a hash of trying to talk to her. She backed away putting the counter between us and asked warily what I wanted. Acutely aware of her reaction I just burbled. Duncan came to the rescue again. With her eye still on me she groped for the vitamin C on the shelf behind her. I was very distressed, I felt that a person working in a pharmacy would meet all kinds of disabilities and would be more tolerant – and it had been the Year of the Disabled only the previous year. How soon people forget.

On the way back to the hospital I realised I had developed a particularly annoying habit. The wording of road signs or advertisements I happened to be passing would stay in my mind and I would repeat them. For instance I would say, 'I hope they put me in the same Freeway South' – meaning 'I hope they put me in the same ward again'. Or 'I really liked the Channel Ten we had at the Sailing Club' – which translates as 'I really liked the fish...'. What made it worse was that I had been unaware that I was doing it until Duncan pointed it out. Just before I made these strange comments I had seen a notice for 'Free Way South' and a billboard for 'Channel Ten' on the free way and incorporated them into what I was saying without noticing they were there. Shauna, when I reported this oddity to her, said my mind was not screening out irrelevant material.

I was unhappy with that first shopping expedition. I vowed I would not go shopping again if that was the reception I would have to expect.

CHAPTER FIVE

If God Could Hear You Now

On the 8th of August 1988 I was fit enough to go to Shenton Park Hospital, an annexe of Royal Perth Hospital. Shenton Park deals with the rehabilitation of patients with head injuries, multiple sclerosis, paraplegia and quadriplegia, strokes and many other disabilities. It has a dedicated staff of physiotherapists, speech pathologists and occupational therapists as well as nurses. For the three to five days before the move I had begun to get bored with the sedentary hospital life at QE11. It says something about the nature of my illness that I had not been thoroughly bored before then. Exhaustion and sleep had been my life up till that point. It had required an enormous effort of concentration to do anything at all – like reading a paragraph from a book or taking a short walk. On one occasion I walked back to the ward from Shauna's office. It was a brisk walk along a corridor then a lift then another fifty metre walk. Shauna came with me so I did not have to blaze my own trail which would have been worse. I was so tired I slept for an hour.

I was aware of some of my limitations by then. In particular I began to very much miss not being able to read. I could manage the physical act of reading. Beyond the blur in my eyes (the left one was much better than the right at this stage) I could see the words clearly enough. That was not the problem. I just could not make any sense of it. I could read the words but the sentence itself baffled me. I used to be a person who could happily curl up with a good book and waste a whole day. So you can imagine my horror at the thought of not ever being able to do that again.

Then there were the limitations of my speech. Dr B said humorously (knowing that I could not argue with his statistics) that in time my speech would be 97.86 per cent of 'normal'. But that did little to cheer me. What did he mean? What was normal? Did he mean the normal me? Or the average normal for my age? Dr B had not known me after all before I had the stroke. Of course I could not ask him about it because I could not formulate the question in my mind. I knew something was troubling me about what Dr B had said but I could not think what. At least that was a merciful thing about my brain, it did not go fretting about things it could not change. In my case it cut out and left those thoughts in the 'too hard' basket. I wanted to ask, 'When will I get my thinking back or my reading?', but I could not do this. I only had the continued certainty that if Dr B could not work miracles at least he was giving it his best effort. I could relax.

Three years after the stroke a doctor said to me, 'You probably won't recover any more now'. I ignored the comment because I already knew that I was making steady progress and that it was not liable to stop just because some person put a limit of years on it. If Dr B had taken that view a few weeks after the stroke, in my immensely vulnerable and suggestible state, I would have believed him and – who knows? - I may have achieved only a fraction of the recovery that I have made. Fortunately nothing like that was ever said to me in the early days. I received only encouragement.

I was apprehensive about going to Shenton Park – and therefore tearful. Yet I could not think of any disadvantages of being moved there. On the contrary I knew they had a gymnasium and the physical work should suit me very well. But I also knew that this step would bring me closer to the real world and I could not imagine how I was going to deal with that when it came. I knew I must not think about it.

At Shenton Park they put me in a two-bed ward and I was to share a room with Rose. 'You'll like Rose', they promised. Rose had battled her way in London in the teeth of World War 11 and she was not going to let a little thing like a stroke stop her now. Rose's left-hand side was paralysed . She did not have the speech problem that I did, she spoke normally. She was a mine of information on strokes. She said, for instance that a third stroke was usually fatal. I managed to say, 'Even a second stroke would be bad enough. I would rather it kill me outright.' Rose was a picture of outraged horror. 'You terrible person!' she said. 'If God could hear you now.' I was no match for Rose, not with my limited speech. I could not answer back and I could not change the subject; I just had to take it. Quite suddenly I knew immense, justifiable frustration!

She told me that patients who did not work hard were soon weeded out of Shenton Park, that there were dozens of people desperate for our opportunity and they would take our place as quick as lightening.

She would not let me help her with anything such as doing up buttons although I was itching to help. She was very worried that although she had passed the physiotherapist's test of walking she might not pass the occupational therapist's test of looking after herself once she was home. She was on tenterhooks the day of that tests. She had been at Shenton Park for six long months. I admired Rose and she was partly responsible for bolstering my sagging attitude.

She and I made cups of tea in the nurses' room. I thought it would be like QE11 where we could make tea whenever we liked as soon as we were mobile. But at Shenton Park we had to be very careful about it so as not to get caught.

Things were very different at Shenton Park and try as I might I could not like the place. There was very little privacy. Rose said that if my stroke had happened in Britain, unless I were very lucky, I would not have had access to the facilities for recovery, that were in Australia. So I really tried to feel I was fortunate. The room I shared with Rose was painted a greyish shade of white. It was high-ceilinged in the way of old houses and sparsely furnished. I had only one tiny cupboard so I sent two-thirds of my belongings home with Alan. The rest - mainly toilet articles, envelopes and a few clothes – were squashed into the cupboard. I had brought detergent as they encouraged us to do our own washing. My clothes consisted of the regulation tracksuit and runners, T-shirts, two pairs of socks, two slippers and a dressing-gown. I felt like a new girl at school.

When I had unpacked I padded down the corridor, socks on my feet, looking for the toilet. A nurse looked at my feet. 'You can't wear those' she said, 'slippers or bare feet'. That rule was to prevent the patients slipping on the vinyl tiles. I chose bare feet.

I did nothing for a whole day. A male nursing aid filled out a form with me and I was intrigued when I was asked, 'Do you feel abnormally cold in winter?' and 'Do you feel abnormally hot in summer?'. I asked the aid why those questions were there. I felt very smug at having asked a question at all but he just looked at me and ignored my question. I found out later that the purpose of those questions was to find out if there was anything wrong with a patient's thyroid gland.

In another wing of the ward there were a few patients who had the sad, slow disease of multiple sclerosis. One of them sang, 'Danny Boy' while he was on the exercise bike. He had a lovely voice and all the wing stopped what they were doing and listened to him. There was applause when it ended.

Everywhere I looked on that first day I saw patients whose reason for being there – disease or accidents – were worse than mine. I began to hate Shenton Park.

A nurse insisted on accompanying me when I took my first shower. I said I had been taking showers by myself for three weeks but she was unimpressed. 'Those are the rules, here' she said primly. But in the end I was quite glad of her. She stopped me leaving the shower without my shampoo, soap, watch, flannel and dressing-gown. She said, 'That is one of the things about a stroke you have to concentrate on every little thing'. I looked at her sharply – that is to say, tunnel vision allowing, I focused on her as best I could with my blurry eye. No, she was far too professional to be implying 'I told you so'.

On the second day at Shenton Park I was seen first by the physiotherapists. Their room had two or three double mattresses scattered on the floor and patients were lying on them. The physiotherapists were moving limbs back and forth with endless patience. The multiple sclerosis patients who came in frequently for treatment, knew the ward's routine and most of the physiotherapists. They bantered back and forth to each other. How I wished I could banter.

I easily placed wooden blocks back in a box with my right hand. Then we went outside for a walk over 'rough terrain'. This consisted of steps up and down and walking up quite steep inclines and on grass and tarmac. It was a lovely day and I enjoyed it. Physiotherapy pronounced me fit so I was able to concentrate on speech pathology.

I was accompanied everywhere by an orderly and in a wheelchair at first, he took me over to the gymnasium. He introduced me to a physiotherapist who smiled at me and said she wouldn't be a minute; then the orderly left. At that moment a boy of about seventeen years was wheeled in. His head was bandaged and shaved and he had metal pieces coming from beneath the bandages. His poor arms and legs were a mass of splints and bandages. He had, I guessed, been in a motor car accident and he was a vegetable. My arm reacted in sympathy and started to tingle. I was convinced I was going to have another stroke and I was rushed back up to the ward to lie down and be seen by the resident. So much for my first day at the gym. I had become very emotional since the stroke as I have said before and although most of my emotional reactions were in the right direction they were over-itensified.

I managed to meet the physiotherapist in the gym the day after. Again I was wheeled down in a chair. I loathed that wheelchair but I suppose it served a purpose: they could not have patients falling over. I enjoyed the gym. I thought, 'I can do these exercises standing on my head, I have been given such simple things to do'. (I had done gymnastics at school). The first exercise I had to do was simple balancing on a 'wobble board' (a low conical board with the point beneath it). For this exercise I had the parallel bars to cling to. I could not balance on it for one second let alone the fifteen seconds as the physiotherapist suggested.

Next were some strengthening exercises on weight machines. I was good at those and could really feel myself becoming stronger especially when the physiotherapist put an extra weight on the machine. By now I could feel that my right side was very weak compared to my left side. But I would stick rigidly to the same weight (although I knew I could be doing more) until the physiotherapist told me to change. It did not occur to me to change the weights myself, that would be making a decision and decisions were much better left to others. I had become very passive. I noticed this in all sorts of ways. I had been a very independent person before the stroke but now I quite happily let others make decisions for me. A combination of my lack of speech and the energy needed for concentration made me accepting of other people's decisions. I needed direction even in simple things.

I had to balance on an upturned bench with a narrow supporting beam, about eight centimetres wide, on its underside. I was supposed to walk along this trying not to fall off the end, then turn around and walk back. My balance was terrible and I fell off all the time.

Next there was the exercise bike and throwing a netball against a wall while standing on a springy board. Then for my concentration the physiotherapist set up a net and she and I played badminton. I could hit the ball quite well at first but as my concentration plummeted, I hit the ball more and more wildly until I had to stop, exhausted. We had been playing for exactly five minutes. Back at the ward I crawled into bed and slept.

A typical day at Shenton Park began with a shower. We all had set times for showers and by then I was showering by myself. I had a mental check list of things that I took into the shower with me. I made myself check no fewer than three times, because I did not want that nurse following me to my room with something I had forgotten. She really had done me quite a favour!

Then we had breakfast. The food was atrocious at Shenton Park but there was not much they could do to make breakfast unpalatable: the cereals came in portion control packets and I did not order toast or the main course. I was surprised there was no low-cholesterol menu. At first I would look at a menu and be unable to register what was written there. Then after a while, I could make a choice if it was between two or three items. I was slow but I saw eventually what it was I was supposed to put down. I stuck to my low-cholesterol diet as far as possible.

A low-cholesterol diet means keeping away from foods containing oil and fat as much as possible, regardless of whether they have cholesterol in them or not. For instance, avocados are sold as 'low in cholesterol' but they are rich in oil. I love avocado but I only eat it rarely now. Meat must be very lean with all the fat cut off. Offal is out and so are chips. Even chips cooked in polyunsaturated oil are off limits because of the oil content. Cheese is terrible and cream, worse. When I had to decide whether to use fat-reduced milk or skim, I chose skim so that I could justify the odd lapse on cheese or cream. The thing I missed most of all was cheese. By the time I left Shenton Park I had lost six kilograms and my cholesterol had dropped to 5.3 millimoles per litre.

Stress I feel coupled with increasing pollution (in our water supplies and food) gives rise to a lot of the illnesses we have today, including stroke. Consider the amount of pesticides in the run-off that pollutes our reservoirs. The same applies to food. Pollutants are in our food whether we are vegetarians or not although there are more in meat. Grazing cows take up the pesticides contained in the vegetation they eat and it is stored cumulatively in their fat. The older the animal the more pollutants it has in its fat.

It makes good sense to follow a low-cholesterol diet. By doing so we not only eat a diet that is good for us but we cut out the cumulative source of pollutants in the fat of meat and the oils of plants (oil is the plant's equivalent of fat). In a strict low-cholesterol diet there should not be much fat intake from any source, animal or vegetable, so the intake of pollutants is less as well.

CHAPTER SIX

Brain Clicks

The saying goes 'Something clicked in my brain'. That is exactly what 'brain clicks' felt like to me, only a hundred times more intense than the feeling I normally associated with that phenomenon. They happened at night while I was asleep and the next day it was as though I had experienced an explosion of knowledge, an enlightenment that had lifted me from one level to another. It was like taking a sudden leap forward and quite suddenly mastering something that had been elusively out of reach. It was a widening of my personal horizons and a sort of, 'I knew that' feeling - a breakthrough.

For example, I had a brain click one night and I woke up to find I could sign my name – something I could not do the day before. It was not until January 1989 that I became aware of brain clicks but when I did I realised that I had been having them over the six months since the stroke. I must have been experiencing them every day immediately after my stroke and I could pinpoint certain milestones in my progress that I now recognised as being the result of brain clicks. Later on they seemed to occur at much less frequent intervals.

At Shenton Park I started the day at 9-30 am with an hour of therapy with Kathryn, my speech pathologist. She noticed that I was leaving the 'the' and 'a' out of my sentences. I found that when a speech pathologist told me where I was going wrong it was a much quicker process of recovery than if I had to wait to discover it for myself. After a session with Kathryn I at least recognised the problem and even if my sentences did not improve at the time they would improve very soon after – probably as the result of a brain click.

I could not get the hang of 'before' and 'after' at all. Kathryn would say, 'Jack got to the ball just before Peter. Who got to the ball first?' It took me quite a few sessions to work that out. Another task Kathryn set me was to turn statements into questions. 'That is the car I bought.' It already looked to me like a question. 'Must not tell Kathryn that', I thought. I finally got some of them right with a good deal of help.

I particularly liked the sessions where Kathryn would talk to me about the mysterious workings of the brain. I came to understand that the more you battled with a problem the more likely the brain was to do something about it.

The undamaged neurons (brain cells) can form new dendrites. A dendrite is like a piece of fine, living cotton that links the cells together. A single neuron is capable of growing one hundred thousand dendrites and there are billions of neurons in the brain. (It is estimated that there are more neurons in a single brain than there are people in the world).

The neurons are linked in networks: the numbers of which defy comprehension.

One of the functions of a neuron is to pass messages from one cell to another. The tip of the dendrite terminates in a structure called a synapse, a slightly swollen area where one cell communicates with another cell. The word for this proliferation of dendrite activity is 'connectivity'. New synaptic connectivity is believed to underlie much of the recovery mechanism and because of connectivity, the brain is able to form alternative pathways around a damaged area. In this way there can be a return of function.

Kathryn told me that the left-hand side of my brain where the stroke had done its damage was where the 'grammar rules' were kept. 'Sequencing' (getting the words in order) also resided here along with the 'vocabulary' and 'sound' centres. No wonder I was having trouble with organising my speech. I had to wait until enough dendrites had formed contacts around my 'sound' centre for me to make words.

I took heart in the fact that I had recovered this far and as far as I knew there was no reason why I could not continue to progress until I was practically back to normal. That was very important to me and I could feel in my bones that one day I would get there.

Other functions of the left side of the brain, Kathryn said were 'writing symbols' and 'reading'. My writing, though never wonderful, had become very bad indeed. I wrote with my left hand at first but even when I managed to write with my right hand the tails of the letters were wiggly and of uneven length. I wrote letters back to front, grouped lower case and upper case letters together and I sometimes missed letters altogether. I could not trust my signature unless I was concentrating hard. It was very trying using my credit card. As well as the doubtful signature, I wrote it slowly as well.

All the damaged left-hand centres in my brain contributed to make difficulties for me in reading. When I read a new word – that is one I knew before the stroke – I knew what it meant intuitively. But although the new word was not lost it was not available to me until that part of the brain resumed working. So I could not, for instance tell people what the book I was laboriously reading was about. In the same way I would listen to and enjoy radio broadcasts but would not be able to repeat any of it to another person.

Kathryn said that 60-70 per cent of speech came from the left-hand side with the rest from the right-hand side of the brain.

The right-hand side of the brain (which, in my case was undamaged) exerted control over 'body language', 'prosody' and 'social conversation rules' as well as 'intonation' and 'emphasis' in order to convey emotion.

At this stage I could not have cared less about my 'body language' if only I could speak effectively. 'Prosody' was a different matter. What was prosody? Kathryn told me it means the 'ability to put words into verse', rhyming. I could for the moment do without that ability too. If only I could swap it for 'sequencing'. 'Social conversation rules' such as being able to take your turn, I did not have to bother about either. I spoke so slowly that by the time I had thought of something relevant to say the conversation had moved on to something else – unless as often happened people waited politely for me to finish. I want to thank my many friends who did just that for me, it must have been excruciatingly tedious for them. 'Maintaining a topic' comes under the right side command. It could have come from my feet, for all the 'topic maintenance' I was able to do. Lack of vocabulary and poor concentration did not help either.

Strokes of the left side and the right side are actually equally represented in a large stroke population but most of the stroke patients that I came in contact with seemed to be paralysed on the left side. That means they were injured on the right side of the brain. They could generally speak quite adequately compared to me. I think some of them at Shenton Park felt I was a fraud to be walking around so well. Lack of a visible paralysis made them think that I was all right. If only I could have told them how dreadful it was not to think beyond concrete realities and not to have a sense of humour. I could not of course, I did not realise it myself. I had my own paralysis.

A few days after moving to Shenton Park Elizabeth came to visit me and said something had happened to my dog, Maggie but that she was all right now. I listened in numb horror to the tale of how Maggie while walking without a lead had leapt onto the road and been run over. She was taken straight to Brendan Kay, the Vet who had been looking after Maggie since she was a puppy. Her back leg was broken and she had a deep skull wound. She was at Brendan's for three weeks. On hearing I was in hospital he only charged me the price of the pin that had to be inserted into Maggie's leg thereby saving me a great deal of worry and money.

Poor Elizabeth she tried to make me see the funny side of it, saying that Maggie had taken herself to hospital in sympathy. Even if I had not entirely lost my sense of humour anyway, I would not have found that joke particularly funny. I reacted quite violently. I cried and went red in the face and I did not care if I was giving myself another stroke or not. The nursing staff try to preserve patients from upsets such as these. Upon arriving in hospital patients are asked whether there are children to be looked after and about pets. Rosemary had told them about my dog and cat, and now this! I calmed down eventually and began to think, 'Maggie is all right so what am I worried about?' But it was a tense moment.

Shortly after I was moved to a larger ward. This was awful. There was not as much room as there had been even in the double room. To make up for it, Mary (one of the patients I met in QE11) was one of the four people in there. I was very pleased to see her again and we quickly renewed our acquaintance. The ward was very noisy with its uncarpeted floors reflecting every sound and with so many visitors for the occupants.

Mary's visitors and my own came in ones and twos, for the other beds it seemed as though hundreds came at once. Eventually I got used to them and Mary and I waited in eager anticipation for the daughter of one patient to arrive from Victoria – we felt we all knew her.

Every night at twelve o'clock one of the patient's needed to be lifted onto the commode. In the semi-darkness, two orderlies and a nurse would appear, throw the curtains round her and switch on the light. It was enough to make one think the Gestapo had come for her. I know the poor thing could not help it but the stench was awful. I would find it hard to go back to sleep. Eventually I would be longing for a cup of tea. Most of us tried to ask the nurses for as little as possible because they were so busy but we were not allowed to make a cup of tea ourselves especially at that time of night. So I just had to ask the nurses – and they would get me one cheerfully enough.

One day about seven weeks after the stroke a group of us were sitting having our coffee on the verandah outside the ward and I looked up at some tall trees. They had been blurred the day before. Now I could see every leaf! That took me utterly by surprise. It felt as though I were dreaming. I tried looking with first one eye closed then the other. My vision was miraculously clear whichever way I looked. I had obviously had a brain click although I had no name for it then. I wondered if by chance my reading had improved too. At that time I was trying to read a book by Len Deighton called *Berlin Game*. But it was as difficult to read as it always had been. I did not realise until much later that Len Deighton writes very complex English. I still found him just as difficult to read even eighteen months later, when I was able to read other less complex books quite well. So I tried to read a magazine but found there was no improvement there either. Some magazines have a very uncomplicated style – and those were the ones I was trying to read – so that particular brain click had not extended to reading.

It was nearly springtime and the weather that year was lovely, bright and warm with none of the searing heat that marks the onset of summer. One day towards the end of August I was sitting outside the ward waiting for Tom to come and see me. Tom visited me every day while I was in hospital.

I was leaning against the rail of the verandah when a man approached me. He was a dwarf, portly, well-dressed in a suit and tie. He wore a hat, thick eyeglasses and carried a briefcase. He peered up at me and touched his hat saying, 'C...C...Could [silence while he grappled with the next word] you show me where ...s...sp...speech th...is?' I answered, 'O...O...Over [but by this time I was flustered and did not remember where it was] you go round...'. He thought that I was making fun of him. He looked sadly at me for a moment and turned away. Fortunately Tom came at that moment and was able to give him the directions he needed. He possibly had aphasia like I did.

I sometimes went to Duncan's for the weekend which was a welcome change from the hospital routine. I no longer bumped into people with my shopping trolley. But a new symptom was emerging. Whenever there was background music playing in a supermarket, I could not concentrate on the shopping – even if I had only two items to buy. It was terribly difficult to keep in mind, for instance 'a tube of toothpaste' until I got to the third aisle if the music was playing. I had to look at my shopping list all the time (yes, I would make a shopping list for two items). Even then I would often have to go back to the begining to collect a bottle of coffee, so thoroughly confused was I by the background music.

It was all very well writing lists but the problem was that unless I had the item itself in my mind, I would miss it. For instance I had to see the 'shampoo' I wanted to buy in my mind's eye (visualise it). If I could see it as a picture of the brand I wanted then I was able to recognise it when I came across it. If I could not do that I would walk right past it with my list and not notice it was there. No wonder every 'new' activity took so much concentration.

Needless to say I never telephoned anybody except in an emergency. But occasionally I called Alan while I was at Shenton Park. He had an answering machine and that made all the difference.

I never used to like answering machines. Like a lot of people it made me cross to hear a cheerful voice telling me its owner was out. And, yes I was one of those people who often did not leave a message at the end of the beep. Alan was the only one of my friends with an answering machine (in 1988). I would ring him up when I knew he was unlikely to be there because I would have ample time to get my message onto the tape without being interrupted. In a normal telephone call the moment someone said, 'Hello?' I was stuck with 'Hello' 'Hello' 'Hello' reverberating round my brain. It would take a while for it to go and the chances were that I would not say, 'Hello' back to them. So they were inclined to say, 'Who's there?' just as I was about to start my, 'Hello'. That would put me off again. I learned to avoid all telephones except Alan's with its answering machine.

After my speech therapy session in the morning came physiotherapy in the gym followed by lunch which was eaten back in the wards. Then we slept or did some washing. Mostly I slept because after I had spent half the morning at speech pathology and half in the gym I was ready to drop. As time went on I used some of the time in the afternoon for reading. I was still trying to struggle through *Berlin Game*, sentence by sentence.

In the afternoon one by one the wheelchairs were pushed to occupational therapy (OT) by the orderlies. I waited for afternoon tea to be brought to the ward and then went to OT myself. The people who had to rely on orderlies to push them around very often missed afternoon tea on the wards and had it in OT when they got down there. If I was really lucky I would have tea twice, my mind was occupied with trivial things such as this. Our day was punctuated by tea breaks and meals.

I felt that the occupational therapist to whom I had been allocated preferred her patients to be more needy than I appeared to be. I could see her lips purse when I brought the typewriter from its place and set it up on the table. The others had to wait for the therapists to do it for them. But my 'independence' was to no avail: the 'how to type' sheets were nowhere to be found and I had to ask for them.

I was given a game to play. I had to make words out of twenty-five letters the same size as Scrabble letters, mounted in a plastic square. I was only aware of about one-third of them. I tried to make the word 'tree' but I could not find any E's. Once having decided on the word 'tree' my mind was reluctant to let go. 'Tree" I said to myself, 'tree...tree...tree'. I shook my head and looked away from the board and looked back. 'Tree?' said my mind hopefully. I took myself in hand with a truly amazing effort, forcing myself to think of another word. I came up with 'there' – not unlike 'tree' but I was thankful enough to have dropped 'tree' at all. Of course that had E's in it too and I could not find an E. The whole thing reminded me of Harry Belafonte's song, 'Got a hole in my Bucket, Dear Liza, Dear Liza'.

When the occupational therapist finally came back and I told her I could not find an E she looked at me strangely and pointed out that there were no fewer than six E's on the board. I could miraculously see them when they were pointed out to me.

I remembered that Shauna had once described this way that I had of dwelling on one word, like 'tree', as an example of my brain's not being able to screen out insignificant trivia. My brain regarded all bits of information as equally important. Even several years after the stroke, if I was tired, I would still be liable to catch the last thing a person said the repeat it. For example when people wished me, 'Happy Birthday' I would respond with 'Happy Birthday to them.

The word game in OT was like the shampoo bottle in the supermarket. Unless I had in my mind what it was I was looking for, I could not recognise it even when I was looking straight at it. That was probably the reason why the board looked as though it was only one-third full to begin with. Somehow I must have remembered some letter shapes better than others.

I joined a game of quoits one afternoon at OT. I had about twenty throws standing about a metre away and I did not get one of them on the pole. I had no idea of how to correct my throw; if it went to the right, I did not throw to the left a little bit the next time and vice versa.

One of the occupational therapists played the guitar. I

thought that playing the guitar would be good exercise for my right hand so I asked Alan to bring my guitar to the hospital. I could not really play before my stroke. I had had a few lessons at one time and another and had given up again when pressure of work or lack or practice became too much. But I thought illogically that now would be a good time to learn. The occupational therapist had a little electronic device that enabled one to tune the instrument but 'playing' my guitar gave me very little pleasure. It became a chore. I did not think about it much at the time but it must have been to do with my disinterest in music generally. At that time I also had a tendency to become intensely agitated about little things that did not matter and I kept myself awake one night worrying that the guitar was going to be stepped on or stolen. So I sent it home with Alan again.

One day I joined in an art class. It was a peaceful retreat from the overcrowded bustle of the OT room next door. The OT room had people in wheelchairs clustered round a table, knitting or playing Scrabble, another group playing quoits and others being persuaded to write or pick up their cup. Next door was different.

The chair-bound art instructor was finishing a painting and invited me to help myself to paper, charcoal and paints. I used to like to paint so I was looking forward to it. I sat gnawing my paintbrush and trying to think about what to draw. I waited; no inspiration came at all. Surely I could draw something? Not a thing came to mind. Maybe I could draw a still life but looking around there was nothing that appealed to me. That should have told me something, there are always stray bottles and brushes, leaves and pine cones around an art room. I accepted the fact that I could not find anything to draw without thinking that it was very likely my condition that was to blame, which it was. The instructor handed me a postcard showing some sheep around a gum tree. So I painted that. I am still intrigued by the thought that, at that time, nothing appealed to me. In a way, it was similar to music. Could my emotional response to music and art – and people – have been impaired? I think that was probably the case. (Later I came to realise my imagination had been damaged by the stroke too). I must emphasise that I did not think of it in this detached way while it was all happening, I just accepted it and did not miss it. Besides there was so much else to relearn.

At the art class I met Paul Berry who was in a wheelchair. Paul held his brush between his big toe and the next toe, somehow resting the handle against the sole of his foot. When he was finished with the brush he put it back in its space, upright in a little rack. Every few minutes he had to rest. The pictures he painted were intricate and lovely – mostly landscapes and seascapes. I was told he had had polio and his hands hung limp and useless at his sides. A few years after I met him, he exhibited his paintings at Burswood Casino in Perth.

Everybody in hospital naturally looks forward to going home. Towards the end of August I was dying to go home. On Dr B's next weekly visit he tested my reflexes, did all the other tests for possible brain activity, listened to my speech and then decided to keep me in one more week. I was downcast. But in hindsight knowing the difficulties I had to face when I was released, even another week in hospital on top of the one he had given me would have been reasonable. I thought of Rose, about her nervousness wondering whether the physiotherapists would pass her as fit to go home. Now I knew what she had been going through.

Another week to stay in the hospital seemed like forever. The weather was still beautiful and OT sessions were conducted outside. Three or four of us would form a circle on the lawn and play Trivial Pursuit. One of the women had Guillain-Barré syndrome. Her illness had begun with a slight cold and she was now paralysed and in a wheelchair. Her speech was paralysed, too. She could move her hands a little and when it was her turn to answer a question she became very excited and gestured her answer. We would interpret for her. She would get better in time, I was told.

One of the occupational therapists found a golf club and some practice balls, the plastic ones with holes in them. I wanted to know if my golf swing had been further damaged by the stroke. From what I could tell from my five of six hits I was doing quite well. Soon I had to stop though as the gardener was frowning – just daring me to dig up a divot.

I stayed the weekend with Margaret just before I left the hospital permanently. Margaret later described my speech at that time as being like two tapes running at the same time. The background tape (inappropriately supplying words from a magazine I had just been reading) would interject in what I wanted to say. It was strange that I was not aware of just how bad I was although I did realise my deficiencies to some extent. I became very exasperated with myself when I could not get some perfectly simple idea across. I would give up the unequal struggle, 'Oh! Shut up' I would say to myself in frustration. It was all there in my head (I thought) so why couldn't I get it out?

Much later I began to realise that what I said was the sum total of what was available to me at the time. I sensed that somewhere in my brain there was a great deal of knowledge stored and that I was just scratching the surface of what was there. That realisation was sinister and sent a shudder down my spine. I was groping to reach words that appeared to be just beyond my grasp. But had I known the full extent of what was locked away I would have been appalled. With each brain click came a further revelation of things that were still lost to me.

That weekend at Margaret's I had what must have been another brain click, part of my reading ability came back. What a thrill it was! I was reading a magazine and quite suddenly it began to make much more sense that it had done previously. Yes, the meaning of what I was reading was still there two paragraphs later. I literally jumped for joy! I no longer stumbled over 'befores' and 'afters' and I could retain the sense of a whole paragraph.

But I was just as stuck as always about numbers. A million meant nothing to me; it might have been ten. We had been concentrating on 'before' and 'after' in speech therapy sessions. I am convinced that helped me to get that part of by brain back in working order more quickly. On the other hand we had not bothered at all with numbers. And my understanding of them had not returned at all.

I constantly visualised my brain, willing it to work again. I thought of it in terms of a 'burnt-out' area (not too big!). Then I visualised little 'mirror' neurons in a different part of my brain being slowly activated – like waking up from sleep. In my imagination I thought of the 'real words and thoughts' as being stored in the area that had been damaged by the clot. But I also believed that these same words and thoughts were duplicated several times (reflected). And the 'mirrors' of these words and thoughts were in other, undamaged parts of my brain and would take over the function of the damaged part in time.

I visualised the area of my speech loss as being supremely

important. As such it had a lot of copies (mirrors) of itself dotted about the brain. 'What I had to eat last night' was of minor importance and probably had one or at most two areas of neurons interested in that type of information. But where I lived was important and required more 'backup mirrors' – perhaps ten. Such visualisation helped me to get to 'know' my brain.

Although I could not use words after the stroke, I could still form mental pictures (picture formation is a right-brain function and I had my damage on the left side). They were not very imaginative pictures and I could not concentrate for long but they worked for me. I could imagine little dendrite extensions growing very slowly from each neuron and little groups of neurons – about six or seven – reaching out their dendrites to other neurons to link up the pathway. The quicker the dendrites grew the sooner I would have my speech back.

At the same time I visualised the blood supply. Blood the bringer of life was giving oxygen and food to provide energy for my precious little neurons. As they woke to the sound of rushing blood I imagined them, wriggling in exuberant excitement towards their task of unlocking the brain. I imagined the dendrites contacting other neurons and with their dendrites they would be forming whole new networks. Then hopefully, there would be what I came to know as a brain click.

At last I was ready to go home. It was the job of the OT Department ultimately to pronounce a patient fit. Some patients who had suffered paralysis had to spend time in a specially built flat. They demonstrated their ability to live independently by looking after themselves here for a day or two prior to going home. I did not have to do that.

My occupational therapist checked my reflexes, how I reacted to a pin pricking my arm, hot and cold, standing on

Abstract representing connectivity

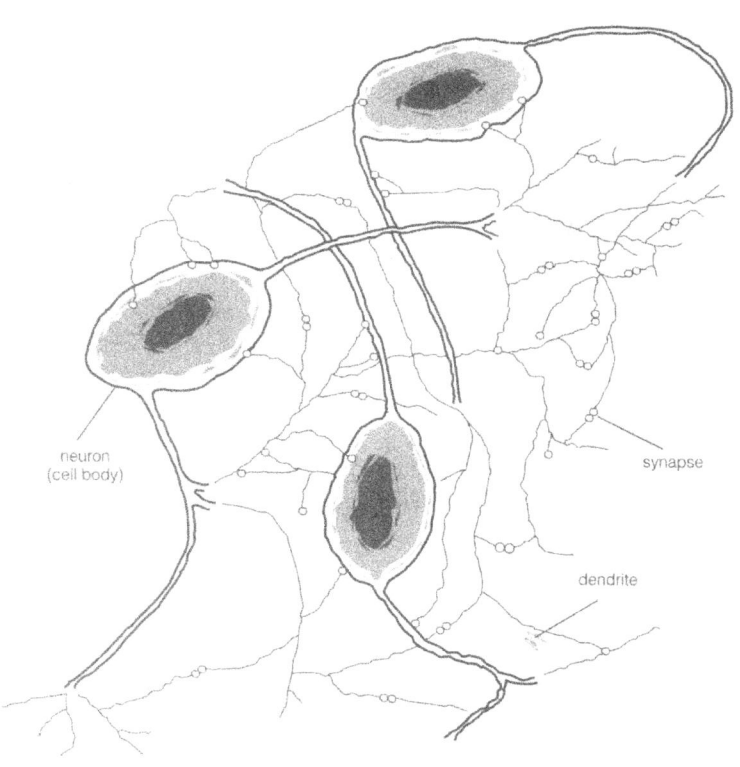

one leg and being pushed. She timed me as I put a set of nails into holes in a wooden board, and eventually pronounced me fit to go home.

After inspecting a display of aids designed to make life easier for people more severely affected (physically) than I was, I was left feeling depressed. There were special knives and forks for people who only had the use of one arm and special ramps and wheelchairs. Except for my speech I was very lucky and did not need these things. I did not even limp very noticeably although I had an awkwardness about my walk. The fact that I did not limp made people I did not know wary of me. The attitude of the pharmacy assistant during my first shopping expedition with Duncan was something I was to encounter many times. I could see them wondering: 'Is she drunk or on drugs? Or just simple?' Friends told me the stroke barely showed – but they knew what was wrong. At the earliest opportunity I would tell strangers of my stroke and I would touch my head. This had a surprising effect on some people. Rosemary saw me doing it one day. She laughed and said, 'You can't do that! Tell them you've been very ill and it's affected your speech, there's no need to touch your head!'. Things were a lot simpler after that salient advice.

The occupational therapist asked if I could write a cheque. I had not tried and knowing what I was like with numbers, I wondered. I had difficulty with the words for numbers. For instance for $87.03 I was unsure whether I was writing $77, $87 or $97 and I was not at all confident of where to put the hyphens in the words. I had to write cheques very slowly – and I thanked my lucky stars for my credit card, which I only had to sign.

My friends Michael and Lynette were very good to me. I was not aware then of what they were doing but they had an air of constancy about them. Michael telephoned me and invited me to stay with them when I left the hospital. I shrank from that. All I wanted to do was go home. But my mind would not formulate the thought – it was too long. The best I could manage was an uneasy squirming on the end of the telephone while I tried desperately to seek order among my scattered thoughts. This resulted in silence from my end. 'Are you still there?' Michael asked. I was puzzled. It did not occur to me until much later that I was just thinking and not saying the thoughts that came into my head.

Michael and Lynette were persevering friends and it is good to have such friends. Even when my mind-sapping timidity sat like a brown cloud around me causing me to refuse their invitations they did not give up on me. Of course I did not know at the time just how unnerving my timidity and shyness were to other people. It was a long time before that occurred to me.

CHAPTER SEVEN

Outward Bound

On 2nd of September 1988 nine weeks after the stroke I was discharged from hospital. I was pleased to be going home at last. At the same time I was nervous to be leaving the comfort of the predictable hospital routine. I was to see Dr B in a fortnight's time.

Dr B viewed his patients with compassion and was marvellous to them although he was sometimes abrupt with visitors and the nurses scurried around when he was due on the ward. He seemed to like dedication in his students and did not appear to suffer fools gladly. I myself tried hard not to appear foolish! But he had his comical side and he would sometimes wink companionably at the patients as he passed the ward.

I relied entirely on him as a way of seeing myself. Listening to what he said gave me the courage to carry on. There were pieces missing in my mind and I needed him to give me direction in trying to reassemble my life. I felt he was the only person who could really know what was going on in my mind and it was a great comfort to know he was there.

Michelle, the student who had been looking after my house picked me up from the hospital. She had Maggie in the car with her and I was shocked to see how Maggie looked. She was grey on her muzzle. She was stiff and awkward (from the pin in her leg). She was shy, uncertain of herself and a most unhappy dog. She was pleased to see me but in a guarded sort of way. I think she thought I would go away again. Perhaps in her way Maggie was reflecting some of my own uncertainties about getting life back to normal.

Not so the cat. Hiraeth was ecstatic. He knew that I was not going away again. Or perhaps cats do not think that far ahead. He brushed himself against Michelle's legs as if to say, 'Thank you for looking after me' and he never left my side for six days. After that he settled down to being his rather arrogant and demanding self.

Hiraeth was pleased to see Maggie after her three-week stay at the veterinary hospital and wanted to play. But Maggie was not in a playful mood. Once Maggie would have chased Hiraeth around the front garden, the cat tail-up in front and the dog a discreet distance behind. Although Hiraeth tried to lure Maggie into the game he had no success and it was another three weeks before Maggie regained enough of her old enthusiasm to play. I suppose her leg bothered her as well.

When I got home I was totally on my own and I moved around the quiet house revelling in my release from hospital. I was quite enthusiastic about cooking low-cholesterol food. At least it would keep me slim. And it appealed to me to have to follow a good diet for the sake of my health.

I could get any food I wanted from the local shops. There was no need to go to the big shopping complexes. If I got stuck these were people I knew, unlike in a large supermarket where one never encountered the same person twice. I had told them early on about my stroke. I wrote a list of things I needed and if I could not find an item one of the assistants would show me where it was. I was still at the stage of having to visualise in my mind the things that I wanted to buy. Gradually shopping became easier. As I bought, for instance tea I found it easier and easier to recognise until I was no longer consciously visualising it at all. Then so I would not have any trouble with change I would offer a twenty dollar note for the tea.

I went twice a week to Shenton Park for my speech therapy sessions. I considered driving my car but decided in the end to go by bus. I knew that I must brave the car sooner or later but later would do. I rang my friend Christine and asked her what buses to catch and she said she would come with me for my first trip. I leaned on Christine a lot. I was on sickness benefits which is a kind of pension and it entitled me to reduced fares. Christine sorted out the fare for me at first. It is difficult on buses. Unless you have the correct fare the driver gets irritable. So offering the driver a five dollar note and waiting for the change would not work. We had to change buses in the city. The driver on the Shenton Park bus was a real sweetie. I am quite sure he would not have minded in the least changing a five dollar note. He helped people on and off the bus and was very good with wheelchairs. I suppose that with a destination like Shenton Park, he knew the majority of us would be on the frail side.

My speech pathologist now was Chris who was responsible

for outpatients. When I first saw her I was suffering from breathlessness in my speech. I kept on forgetting to take a breath sufficient to finish a sentence. This was because of concentration again. I was trying so hard to keep in mind what I was going to say that I had literally no time to breathe. I would be gasping at the end of a sentence. The problem was that my sentences had become longer. Imagine having to learn to breathe again. Chris gave me breathing exercises that helped a little but what helped most was when I breathed as if I had a song to sing. I tried to breathe every three or four words and that appeared to help me until my normal breathing patterns returned. The breathlessness lasted about four months.

The trip to Shenton Park became a real nuisance and I asked Chris if I could attend sessions at a hospital nearer to my home. It was arranged and thereafter I went to Bentley Hospital in the Perth suburb of Bentley.

Chris suggested that I also join a group that she ran at Shenton Park. This group had outings and not just sessions of speech pathology. This was a lovely idea. The group did all sorts of things and the members nick-named it the 'Outward Bound Group.' They had just been to the Casino in Perth when I joined them and they were planning a visit to the Art Gallery next.

I was to meet the group for the first time on Friday the 16th of September. The group members – Wally, Jean, Yvonne, Ken and Audrey – were all in various stages of speech aphasia, like me. Towards the end of the first session something came to me in a flash of recognition. These were the same people that were in the 'mind picture' I had had just after the stroke and which had given me so much hope when I had lost all powers on speech. Audrey was just getting up to go (which she had been doing in the dream) and the others were in the exact places that they occupied in the dream. I told them excitedly about it. Jean and Yvonne were very interested but Wally, a former engineer was sceptical. But whatever it was (Carl Jung speaks of 'messages from the angels' when this sort of thing happens to us) it was a great comfort to me at the time I had the dream and I have my own views about it.

I wondered when it would come: the boredom, the loneliness, the depression. One day I woke up and it was there – a feeling of despair and emptiness. My disabilities were so real. I did not spend all that time in hospital just pretending I was ill. The disabilities were all mine and not a thing anyone could do would make them any better.

Another thought that I kept quietly hidden was 'What about my job?'. I finally faced that one. The answer was: 'Even if I do ever get my speech back I'll probably have another stroke from the stress of it all particularly if I try teaching again. So what about a different job altogether'? That is where I would break down and cry. I was sure I would not be able to work at all that I would moulder on the pension forever, unwanted – and that would fuel my tears anew.

I could not even read books for pleasure. The ones I could read were so simple that the content did not really interest me.

When I had visitors in hospital it was very pleasant and rounded off the day nicely. There I had not suffered from loneliness or even boredom or depression. It was a very structured day and I was happy in the company of other patients. If visitors did not come for a while I magnanimously forgave them and watched the television instead.

Things were very different at home. If I expected visitors and they did not come I brooded. If they were late I fumed or, depending on my mood burst into tears. Needless to say I expected someone to call every day. Had I ever had callers every day in the past? Of course not. I could not help my murderous look when I opened the door to a friend, bright and breezy, talking about work.

I had nothing to contribute. I could not read a newspaper; it was too tiring. I listened to talks on the radio all day (thank you Radio National and 6WF – I wonder how many other people's sanity you have helped to save) and could understand them quite well but needless to say I could not discuss them. Before I had uttered two words I was floundering. My visitor would sit politely perhaps offering a word to help me out. And I was petulant enough to think that they did not come and see me often enough! I ought to have been ashamed of myself but I really did not know how very difficult it was for them. At that time half an hour with me must have left my them drained. Poor things!

Eventually I had to take antidepressants. Naturally I did not want to go to a doctor, when one is depressed, one does not want to do anything. But I was whisked off to the doctor by Yvonne, a nursing sister – and there was nothing I could do about it. The doctor made the mistake of sympathising with me. He said, 'If my circumstances were like yours I would feel depressed too'. My lip quivered. Yvonne quickly grabbed the prescription and bundled me out. I took the antidepressants for some months and I felt quite a lot better.

In mid-September I was subject to strange and rather frightening turns particularly at night. They reminded me of the angiogram, the palpitations were the similar. When they happened I breathed deeply and stared at the ceiling in fright. They never lasted more than thirty seconds but that seemed like an eternity. Yvonne said, 'When anything like this happens, call me'. But I did not like to especially when I was still alive at the end of a turn. It seemed unnecessary and besides – I did not want to 'cry wolf' for every little thing. On the whole I preferred to know which of my symptoms were real and which were imagined.

That attitude was not as reckless as it sounds. After all Dr B had said that I was most unlikely to suffer another stroke from this clot. I was taking aspirin religiously and hoping it was keeping my blood 'thin'. I was glad I had decided not to panic about the 'turns' because all manner of things happen, Dr B told me as the body readjusts itself. It seems that as the nerves 'switch on' they go through a 'faulty' period. For example my eyelid started twitching about five times an hour even when I was not tired. I was just about to tell Dr B about it when the twitching stopped. It was as though, in the brain, reconnection to the muscle in the eyelid had to go through a settling down period. I applied the same logic to the palpitations. When I reported them to Dr B on my next visit he sent me to a cardiologist who wired me up to a portable heart monitoring machine for twenty-four hours. There was nothing wrong.

A day of eerie quietness dawned on 11th of September. I was uneasy. Trying to shake the feeling off I went into the garden to peg out some clothes. The trees were motionless, dogs were quiet and the birds were not singing. There was a grey cast to the sunlight shining on the fence and brickwork. I stood there for a few moments the towel I had draped around my neck slowly seeping water through my T-shirt. An icy cold shudder gripped me: it was obvious, I had had another stroke while I was asleep. It had affected my ears. Slowly I tested my limbs. My right arm was all right the fingers still worked and nothing was obviously wrong with my right leg. My squinty eye was no worse than usual. Upon closing one eye and then the other, while looking at a leaf I was able to ascertain that fact.

Then what was it? Of course it was an eclipse. I had not

heard anything about an eclipse but I was sure it was either that or the beginning of the end of the world. On the whole I felt I would settle for an eclipse.

I missed the news that night and had to wait until the next day to find out whether in fact there had been an eclipse or not. I was not going to bring the subject up. I had been so worried that I had looked up at the sun and seen it eclipsed; now if I ever recovered from the stroke I would have detached retinas to contend with. Finally Margaret said the magic words, 'Did you see the eclipse yesterday?'. I said nonchalantly, 'Oh, yes'. Fortunately my retinas were intact.

There were times when I did panic. On 27th of September Yvonne rushed me to QE11 when I had a tingling sensation in my right arm and hand. I was WORRIED! I was quite sure I was having another stroke. I had a pain in my chest too. Fortunately I could not get through too many emotions – I was just stunned. A wretched resignation took over. But I was certainly worried. Yvonne and I arrived at the Casualty Department and she steered me through the red tape and into a queue of people waiting to be seen by a resident. I stayed very quiet. The real reason for my relapse was beginning to dawn on me. I was very meek and only wanted to get away. When the doctor said the pain around the heart was a pulled muscle – I knew! Back in the car again I admitted sheepishly to Yvonne that I had been polishing my van. The effort had been too much for me. It was a long time before I got used to the idea that my right side had been considerably weakened.

John, whom I met at a country ram sale some time before the stroke, was often at Shenton Park visiting his mother and he used to visit me as well. He had promised that when I was discharged from hospital, he would take me out to dinner. He was as good as his word and rang me up soon after I was released, at a time when I could barely speak on the telephone. 'Would you like to come out for tea?' 'No' I replied 'yes I'd like to'. I was still mixing up 'yes' and 'no'. We went to a very pleasant fish restaurant where I stuck to my diet absolutely. Only the most boring of foods remain when you seriously follow a low-cholesterol diet. No chips, no ice cream – I even took my coffee black because they did not have skim milk. What a bore! In spite of that John later asked me out to see a film. We saw *See No Evil, Hear No Evil*, a comedy but I had lost my sense of humour. I laughed politely when I thought John was looking at me but I was completely unaware that my sense of humour was missing; I just thought the film was silly. I began to have an inkling of this loss after talking to my neighbour, Vonny. She told me she had had a small stroke and it had affected her humour as well. We swapped stories of laughing at only the most obvious jokes. If a joke was too long it lost us altogether. It would be a long time before I could tell a joke of my own.

John was valiant. He took me somewhere every second weekend either to the cinema or out to dinner. And once I went down to his farm for the weekend. It is a magnificent place; the homestead is old with high ceilings and a beautiful verandah. I had forgotten John told me he used to race cars. We set off fast over the paddocks in a jeep which was scary enough for me. We left the road suddenly to inspect a flock of lambs and went so close to them that I could have leaned over and touched one. And then when we came to a steep hill John just drove the jeep straight at it. My eyes widened in horror – I have a phobia when it comes to heights – I screamed and kept my eyes tightly shut until we stopped on top of the hill. That was stress.

Before I had the stroke I had booked and paid for a holiday

in England at Christmas time. I was going to see Ben and my mother. There really did not seem to be any reason why I could not still go. Dr B said that by December I would be fit enough. So I had from September when I came out of hospital, until then to make myself ready.

CHAPTER EIGHT

Ledges

Strokes can occur at any age although they are more frequent in the seventh, eighth and ninth decades. In the hospital although the majority of people were in the older age group there were some younger people as well. One of the aspects of stroke that made it particularly devastating for us was the interruption to our working lives.

At the time of my stroke my whole livelihood depended on my career and I foolishly did not have 'loss of income' insurance. I simply had not thought of losing my job through illness or any other cause. While I was in hospital the occupational therapists had tried to help me find employment but it became obvious that all the things they came up with required too much concentration for me. To work in a shop, for example would be quite impossible when I could not even do my own shopping, particularly if there was background music. And giving change would be quite beyond me. It is surprising how many jobs involve numeracy. I would be hopeless working in a garden. Just imagine if I were given a patch of soil ten metres long and asked at what intervals I would sow ten plants?

One day I made an embarrassing mistake at an ATM. I deposited some notes that I had counted and recounted – and counted again just to be on the safe side. I entered them in the machine as $90. A day or two later I received a curt letter from the bank telling me that the safe had been opened with three people present and there was only $80 in the envelope. I came to the conclusion that I had thought there was $90 in my hand and no amount of checking and rechecking could budge me from that figure.

So I arrived home without the prospect of a job to go back to. To make things worse I had planned for some years to take up romance novel writing. Now suddenly I had all the time to do it in but my brain did not have one idea. I thought that even if I could not write it down surely I could get the ideas together. But my creativity was entirely non-existent. I was reminded of Jean in the Outward Bound Group. Jean was an artist by profession. After the stroke she had picked up her brush from time to time only to put it down again in disgust. She could not think of anything to paint. The group would encourage her, 'Start with a tree' someone said. But we all knew the difficulty although none of us could express it. You need your emotions intact and in contact with your thinking to be able to paint. Jean did eventually start to paint again about three years after her stroke.

It is hard to describe this detachment of emotions and

thinking. Imagine your brain is split into five parts (due to the stroke) each entirely separate from the others. Before the stroke these parts of the brain were linked together but now there seems to be no connection between them. Yet each individual part seems to be functioning quite adequately.

Imagine now that each brain-part is responsible for some process (a function that is not done in the other four parts). One part is devoted to the 'Emotions', one to 'Thinking', one to picture-making or 'Visualisation', another to 'Speech' and yet another to 'Movement' for the control of the paralysed arm or leg.

Everything you see and hear goes into the appropriate part of the brain. For example music goes to 'Thinking', 'Emotions' and 'Visualisation'. But it goes straight in – so that you no longer enjoy it! It is as if you are watching the notes go up and down in 'Thinking'. Very little is received in 'Emotions. You can see them in your mind's eye playing drums and flutes in 'Visualisation'. But the whole lot does not come together and is therefore pointless.

Now you would like to talk about the music or wave your arms about conducting it. You have to get the thoughts from their separate parts to the part labelled 'Speech' in order to talk about it or to 'Movement' in order to conduct. You can imagine the massive organisation of the different areas involved (juggling each one individually) as well as the concentration that would be required for that exercise. In my case it could not be done.

But in spite of all that the brain is working overtime on its own recovery. Soon it is able to do it. It just takes a little time to grow back the network of dendrites. In Jean's case when this happened she was able to paint again.

I knew that I must prepare myself for work again somehow.

I did not have much paralysis. But I felt that overdoing things would set me back even further. So I started in an easy way by driving my van. Unfortunately the choke was faulty and this made driving difficult. It seemed to be stuck in the full-on position and the van would roar up to the corner of the street and wait there revving and moving forward slightly – so much so that I had to put my foot on the brake. Its petrol consumption was enormous too. I tried to have it fixed but each time I left it at the garage it would be all right for a while and then another problem would surface. And I found it excruciatingly hard to take it to the garage in the first place.

First I would have to telephone to make an appointment. A voice would reply, 'Crisafio's'. I would take a run at it – not too many words you understand, for fear of not completing the sentence - 'Th...th...the car doesn't go'. I could not give my name or I would forget what I had rung for. Understandably I loathed telephones. There would be a short pause perhaps generated by my abruptness. I knew I had been abrupt to the point of rudeness but I thought miserably there was nothing I could do about it. Charlie and Tony Crisafio were very understanding, it did not take them long to realise who it was. I gave them no clues and they had to try to find out themselves what was wrong with the car.

The engine also played up gleefully. It took its time to start particularly when it was cold until the poor battery was almost flat. It rushed along when it did start and then stopped suddenly, rather like riding a horse. Why on earth didn't I ask one of my friends to help? It did not occur to me. I doubt whether anybody was aware of the difficulties with the car at the time. I just could not communicate the most obvious things. If somebody had said to me, 'That choke sounds rough,' it would almost certainly have brought it to my mind – 'Yes, of course there's a problem – in fact it's been irritating me come to think of it ever since I came home. Why didn't I think of that?' Although I had a picture of the choke in the 'Visualisation' part of my mind and because I was irritated by it, it had entered the equally isolated 'Emotions' centre, it did not go into the 'Speech' area where I could have done something sensible about it. I put up with the problem for eight months.

It did not take me very long to readjust to driving. At first everything about the car – except the steering wheel for some reason – was unfamiliar. I had forgotten which way the gear shift went for reverse or the forward gears. I was uncertain which pedals to press. Fortunately the OT people had warned me about driving at night or when it was raining. I think putting the windscreen wipers on or the lights, would have been the last straw. But it was not like learning to drive all over again thank goodness. Once I had worked it out and had used the controls I did not forget them again. I was nervous at first and drove rigidly with all of my muscles tense. Mainly I was frightened of losing concentration when I ventured too far from home. Accordingly I made my first trips to the local shops; then to a shopping complex about four kilometres away. Then, full of daring to a shopping centre eleven kilometres away called Booragoon.

Getting to Booragoon was all right. But I was so drawn from the concentration required that I could not do any shopping. After a short rest I went straight home. I was a bit shaky but managed to make the distance without having to stop.

The next thing I attempted was the trip through the centre of Perth to Shenton Park. This involved quite a difficult turn-off from the freeway where several lines of traffic had to be crossed. I concentrated hard and set off. The earlier expeditions had put me in good stead. I was no longer fumbling for the gears and even the terrible freeway turn-off seemed easy. It was a quiet time of the day to make the trip between the morning and lunchtime rush periods. Once I had done it successfully the first time I had no further problems.

I was still confused with right-hand side and left-hand side. These would cause difficulties for a long time yet. I knew which way to turn to get to a place but saying 'Turn right' or 'Turn left' confused me. I also had problems with red and green lights but I was well aware if this. I would look at each light with the fixation of a chicken and will it to divulge its secret, whether I was to go on or stop. Very soon I got the idea.

Red and green lights must have been one of those areas waiting for me to work on in terms of brain clicks. Sometimes in speech therapy we would work on an aspect of speech or awareness and often, even the next day I would have control over it. We had not studied the significance red and green lights on one's driving ability and it took me a week to do it by myself. I felt with a speech pathologist's help, it would not have taken so long. It seemed that I needed to know that a certain thing was wrong before my brain began to work on it.

Another problem with driving was that I had to think about staying on the left-hand side of the road, instead of just doing it. It is quite a weird feeling but I got over that very quickly. If I drove with no distractions – certainly without the radio – I very soon began to relax.

In early October I had a scare when my lymph glands swelled up on either side of the carotid artery. That is the one leading up through the neck to the brain – the one that was blocked before. The more I thought about it and the the more I put my hand up to touch the little nodules the more convinced I was that they had a sinister meaning. As well as that I had a tingling sensation in my right arm again and my lip was curling

– I was a mess! I was going into Shenton Park that day and I decided to ask them if I was going to have another stroke.

On my way there I began to feel better as realisation dawned on me. I had used dental floss on my teeth and my lack of coordination made me quite savage at times without meaning to be. So I could have damaged the gum. That was quite likely to have set up a slight infection in turn affecting the lymph glands. I spoke to a doctor who reassured me that I was all right.

I was gradually beginning to see the tingling sensation and the lip curling as favourable signs, that the nerves were finding their way and beginning to belong to new networks. There were bound to be hiccups.

I was becoming a lot more aware of my limitations and they got me down. I had noticed before, in an oblique sort of way that I had very little in the way of a sense of humour. Now I grew really worried about it. It may seem that for someone who could not speak much this should not have mattered. But without a sense of humour life is very flat. We were asked once at school to write down the three things that were most important to us. Almost to a person we put 'sense of humour' as one of the three and many put it first. Now I am in the unenviable position of knowing exactly what it feels like to lose my sense of humour.

It is what we use to entertain friends and to get out of awkward situations. It helps to make a joke when we are at a party. But more than that when our sense of humour is in good order we have a sense of internal well-being. After I regained some of my sense of humour I began to notice the little things. One day for example, down at an Italian growers market the few people that were in the shop stopped and listened as an Italian woman threatened, in Italian, to disembowel the proprietor. At least that is what it sounded like. She may have been commenting on the nice day but I did not think so. The proprietor answered with asperity, finished weighing her apples and turned round beaming at another customer. Nobody laughed but judging from the looks of interest on people's faces we had all been entertained. That is the sort of scene I had been missing, something supremely unimportant yet adding to the variety of daily life.

On a radio broadcast one day I listened to a professor talking about an addiction study. He said that people have always tried deliberately to change the plane of their mind through alcohol, exercise or drugs. He went on to say that sensory deprivation was a torture that could drive a person mad. The loss of humour and with it, variety, was my personal 'sensory deprivation'. Even though I had been aware of the loss of my sense of humour before - and had even experienced some slight recovery of it. It was not until ten months after the stroke that the full impact hit me. When this happened I was left with such a sense of loss that I might well have taken to alcohol, drugs or even exercise to add the variety my life lacked and to change the plane of my mind. I knew that I had once experienced a life different to this one, where I had taken richness and colour for granted or as my due: and now I was left with this, where nothing changed and nothing interested me much. Fortunately it was just three weeks that I had to spend in this limbo before another brain click occurred and I felt more humour in my life.

Of course I still had my 'feeling' or 'emotional' world unconnected as it was (or seemed to be) to other parts of my mind. Which so often consisted of just tears and nothing much else and who wants to cry while watching the Olympic Games on television? - especially if one has to ask, 'What tune are they playing?'. I recognised the tune but could not put a name to it (it was 'The Star-Spangled Banner'). I did not even save my tearfulness for the Australian or British teams. I cried when anybody won.

Many people who have had a stroke are tearful and easily upset. Purely from my own experience it did not mean that I was upset just because I cried a lot or that I was more in touch with my emotions. In fact my emotions seemed a bit superficial, elusive: 'Tears, idle tears, I know not what they mean...' (Tennyson). Once I had reduced myself to tears I felt pretty silly about it and then I had a reason to cry. Of course there are plenty of legitimate reasons to get upset but a silly thing like watching the Olympic Games is not one of them. I know I had felt just as much (if not more) before the stroke and I had not been reduced to tears then. On my annual visit to see Dr B I mentioned that I had this problem. 'Well,' he said laconically, 'you deal with it with the British stiff upper lip.'

A little of my sense of humour came back in October 1989. I made a 'joke'! It was a one-word joke and I cannot remember what it was about but I remember the occasion vividly. Yvonne and Mike were taking me to see the ice-skaters Torville and Dean at the Perth Entertainment Centre. They were very encouraging. I had not been in any crowded place since my illness and I was a bit unnerved by it. There was not much time before the show we had a quick drink and then took our seats round the ice. It was a relief – the comforting darkness of the stadium and not having to talk to anybody. I just relaxed and enjoyed it. The two skaters come from my home town of Nottingham so I particularly wanted to see them. Afterwards we drove straight home. It was so nice when friends went to the trouble of organising things for me. It could not have been much fun for them with me being the way I was.

The return of a rudimentary sense of humour was, oh so slight but definitely there: the result I know now of another brain click. At the same time my handwriting became easier and my speaking more fluent. I was writing letters every week to Ben and my mother so it was easy to see a sudden breakthrough. It was as though I had been lifted physically onto a higher level, it happened so suddenly. It was like magic or a miracle. Sometimes it was like climbing the steep face of a mountain. I would try for three to four weeks thinking about the dendrites linking up and growing rapidly but nothing seemed to be happening. But I knew I was moving slowly up the mountain – and perhaps those dendrites only had an infinitesimal way to go before they linked hands with a dendrite from another neuron and a whole new thought process could take place. I considered that to be a 'ledge' in my 'mountain-climbing' analogy. There would be a rest (days, weeks or months) where nothing appeared to be happening and then up I would go again.

CHAPTER NINE

Rip Van Winkle

I was still having trouble reading certain things. When John took me out to dinner I had to ask him to read the menu to me and let him help me with the decision of what to eat. Menus were especially difficult to read and decisions were still as hard as ever to make. Sometimes on menus it was their large writing and even spacing (so that the printing and the spaces between were the same size) that were the problem. I also could not keep the required amount of information in my head in order to make a choice. So John would help me.

I had noticed this problem I had with reading large print months before when I was still at Shenton Park. We had a final year speech pathology student who had come to do part of her practice at the hospital. She had held up cards for me to read. The type had been enlarged so that it was almost exactly the same size as the spaces between the lines. I took one look, the words ran together and I could not sort them out at all. I asked her if it was a trick. She said, blushing, 'Not at all. I thought it would help to make the letters big.'

One day I set about cleaning out my filing cabinet. Deeds to the last house I had owned went into the rubbish bag as well as old and some new insurance policies and instructions for equipment I no longer owned, and some I did. There were driving licences going back years. The trouble was that I could not relate to the year on them: 1980 meant as little to me as 1988. So I threw them all out. It was as though years had lost all meaning for me. I could read 1985 but the significance was lost on me. I did not know if 1986 was before or after that date and I certainly did not care. Unencumbered by trivial things like dates I just threw them out. I was about to start on my tax file when my accountant friend Alan called in and stopped me.

It was the same with months. Although I could list the months in order from about three weeks into my illness, one month did not mean more than any other. I could quite happily say my birthday was in July when in fact it was in June. I knew the names were month names but the significance of the passage of a 'month' of time eluded me.

I was talking to a friend, Mandy who worked in her spare time for a firm that specialised in filling in tax forms. She was surprised that so many people had to come to her with tax forms when they could easily fill them in themselves. She said some people have trouble with any form at all. I could identify with that.

I had always filled in my tax form myself in previous years, I had had hardly anything to claim and therefore it was easy.

Every form has a space for one's name; I found that at last and wrote my name in it. The form swam in front of me. When it settled I was gazing at the space marked 'tax file number'. I knew that I had difficulty with numbers so I laboriously transferred the number one digit at a time. By the time I had got the group certificates in the wrong order and had used correction fluid on a dozen items on the page I was ready to swear. Alan called round to see me. 'I said I'd do your tax for you', he grumbled. I gratefully handed it to him. Maybe Mandy's clients have a similar problem. If so I sympathise with them. Whenever I looked at a form the questions did not seem to bear any relationship to the spaces for the answers – even if I knew the answers.

I was becoming sorry for myself. I shunned parties and even acquaintances whom I did not know well. I would see only my closest friends – and these I wanted to see as often as possible. I never went out on my own in crowds, they bothered me. And I began to feel neglected. It was hard, very hard. If only I could have kept myself occupied. Even then reading was out of the question, I still could not manage much more than a page of easy reading without becoming tired because of the concentration involved. I went back to *Berlin Game* periodically to see if I could read it yet. The answer was always, 'No'. I had a feeling that once I could read this book without difficulty I could read anything. At the same time I avoided anything to do with biology or chemistry, the subjects I used to teach. I knew instinctively that I could not manage them.

Maggie and I went for walks around empty streets devoid of people. There was not even another dog to be seen. I would arrive back at my empty house depressed, flinging myself into a chair and thinking, 'What now?'. The silence was driving me mad.

In this period I would see a friend perhaps once a day for half an hour or so. I had become well aware of my shortcomings – too well aware. I wished I could go to sleep, like Rip Van Winkle and dream away the rest of my recovery and wake up to find myself whole again.

To put it bluntly my friends had to put up with my being very dispirited, with no imagination and with a rudimentary sense of humour. When they made a joke it fell flat because I could not understand it. I could not even say words to the effect of 'Hang in there, it won't be that much longer now' – I did not have the imagination. My sense of reaching out to people was totally inactive: therefore I could not make friends and keep friends. Although I knew I was boring beyond belief I could not say that I knew it. No comforting words ever came to mind.

Fortunately before my friends could start doing the thing I feared most – gradually not seeing me at all – I decided to do a 'Rip Van Winkle' of my own. I wanted to disappear from view for a while, to rely on myself instead of my friends – and to do that I needed to find something to occupy my time. I had until December to fill in before I went to England and Dr B said I should be able to work again 'in the New Year'. I had a typewriter and decided that now would be a good time to learn to type properly.

On the 17th of October I started a two-week typing course run by the Commonwealth Youth Support Service (CYSS, now 'Skillshare'). I recommend typing to anyone who has had the same type of stroke as I had. It does wonders for the concentration.

There were six in the group. None of us currently had a job so we were doing the course while we waited for something to happen. One of my fellow students was Sunil, a Sri Lankan accountant whose family were soon to be following him to Australia. I became friendly with Sunil. In the preliminary chat with the instructor about how much experience we had had in typing I said I had done some typing, a fortnight's course at a 'Sight and Sound' school twenty years before. At the end of the Sight and Sound course I had reached twenty-five words a minute.

It was wonderful having to be somewhere every day, on time for my class. It added texture to the day. I enjoyed the company of the acquaintances I met when we stopped a couple of times for coffee and the conversation around me was pleasant. No one appeared to notice my funny way of talking after a while. So the course was a very nice interlude in my long struggle to get better.

The first two days I nearly collapsed with exhaustion. We typed for three hours with a couple of breaks and we had access to the typewriter, if we liked in the afternoon after the class had finished. I was confused: I could not understand where the other members of the typing group were getting their 'fingering' (where to place their fingers on the keys) from. I knew the fingering already from my earlier lessons but how did the others know what to do? The instructor had not told us and there were some brand new typists among us. It was a puzzle. I looked at the sheet we had been given. No clue there. Then I tried to visualise what the fingering looked like – and there it was on the sheet in front of me! This was another example of 'not seeing the shampoo on the supermarket shelf' or the E's in the game.

Ten minutes after we started I developed a dreadful headache. I stopped what I was doing, pecking at the D key and talked to myself. If the others had not thought I was odd before they certainly would have done so now if they could have heard what I was thinking. I said to myself 'so you think you'll give me a headache? It may be another stroke but it's much more likely to be my body reacting against the inordinate amount of work that has been flung at it in the last ten minutes.' In spite of the headache, I persevered for the whole three hours. It did not get any worse and it went away completely when I went home. It was just the concentration again.

I was glad I had taken myself in hand like that. The next day the headache was back again but it was not so severe and it disappeared after that. For the remainder of the course I was clear of headaches but I was fully aware of the amount of concentration that the typing needed and felt very tired in the afternoon. I would sleep then.

I was astounded by the progress I made after I started typing. My speech and even my handwriting improved after four days. I began to join my letters together in handwriting.

I had a new speech pathologist, Suzanne at Bentley Hospital. She encouraged me to carry on with the typing. I made another big step forward, I actually complimented her on her grasp of my situation. I had not been able to say anything remotely complimentary before that. This then was a real milestone: to be able to see something from another person's point of view, however limited.

I found that from about the fourth day I could type without being too disturbed by other people typing. My concentration had improved markedly. That in turn led to my being able to talk in a crowd of two or three people, usually without losing my train of thought. Before it had been very difficult for me to contribute to a conversation. For example if somebody started talking about Nottingham I might want to say, 'Torville and Dean come from Nottingham'. But because I was so slow someone would leap in with something about the Nottingham

Forest football team. By this time I would have completely forgotten what I was going to say. If someone remembered that I wanted to say something that was when I would say, 'Oh! Shut up' in disgust at myself. I would feel so frustrated! But after the typing course I grew a lot better at keeping in my mind what I wanted to say.

As well as helping my concentration the typing was good for my right hand. It ached and twitched after a session of typing but I would take a paracetamol tablet at night and the pain would be gone by morning. After a week, it disappeared altogether.

One of the difficulties I had with typing was getting my finger to press down on the typewriter keys. I would find C and my finger would be on the key and ready to press – but I could not do it. It was a case of 'visualisation' blocked on it's way to 'movement' again. Sometimes I would physically lower myself to typewriter level in my efforts to make the recalcitrant finger press the key, and it would not. Then, at last slowly the finger would press the key and C would appear on the page. I had to go through the same thing for all the other letters and the more tired I became, the longer it took me. This happened with my left hand as well as my right.

The day came for our first test. I could read the words that we had to type on a piece of paper but I found it very hard to type 'Jenny' at the top of the sheet. I took so long typing my name that I considered writing it out in longhand on paper so I could copy the letters in type. I found I could not ignore the other people typing. Every so often I would link up the key in my mind with the pressing of the finger and 'Bingo!' I had made another letter. There was the clacking of typewriters all around me, people typing furiously and me punctuating the cacophony with one key every now and then. I could not be upset, could I? I was doing my level best – but it was all quite surreal. I wanted to laugh!

When it was time to add up the mistakes we had made I found I had not made many. I was just slow. For those unfamiliar with how the tests work, the number of words typed in five minutes are counted. The number of words are divided to give the number of words per minute and the number of mistakes are subtracted from the final figure. I had made only three mistakes but I had no idea whether I was adding or subtracting the words. 'Ninety words per minute', I announced after I had been calculating long after the others had handed theirs in. The instructor checked. 'Four words per minute', she said. The others beamed at me. 'We didn't think you would do so well' they said!

Sometimes there were words spelt the American way on our prepared typing sheets. I set about changing them to our way of spelling. Could I think what to do with 'center' to make it 'centre'? I tried the tried. Somewhere in the brain's 'word processing' division I knew exactly what to put. My spelling was fine. I had even been able to spell 'beautiful' on the thank you letter I had sent my former students when they sent me flowers in hospital. No, that was not the problem. I timed myself; it took me three and a half minutes to change 'center' to 'centre'.

So what was the problem? I could see the word 'centre' in my 'Visualisation' compartment very clearly. It should have gone straight to 'Thinking' and thence to 'Movement'. But the prepared typing sheets, with the spelling 'center' bypassed 'Visualisation' – and once I had got one thing in my mind it was hard to replace it with anything else.

I met Helen, a friend of Alan's in October. Even though I was not conscious of it at the time making friends with Helen did an enormous amount of good for my confidence and self-esteem. Helen was willing to be friends in spite of my illness even though I was not myself in so many ways.

To start with I was painfully timid with Helen. We get used to having our say in conversation within very exact limits ('turn-taking' as the speech pathologists call it). If we have not said what we plan to say within moments of the opening being presented to us we may as well not have our say. Sometimes with me there would be a gap of as much as five seconds before I could reply. Count that to yourself the next time you are in conversation and you will see what I was up against. Consequently I got quieter and quieter. Helen did not appear to be fazed by this, she chatted on quite happily herself. It was very restful.

I had little time for children at that time and Helen had ten year old twin girls. They were delightful children, friendly and helpful. But I was battling to deal with one person then and I could not concentrate on more than one person. Time after time I had to stop myself becoming agitated when they, or any other children were around. It is possible that they so much reminded me of the particular stage that I was going through that I thought of them as competition.

I found it impossible to say that I was pleased or that I enjoyed people's company. I realised this at the time but no matter how hard I resolved to say pleasant things to people I would always come unstuck particularly when I was tired – and that was nearly all the time. I was all right when talking about what we might have for lunch. Or if we went shopping I could pick up some oranges and put a name to them. But back home when I tried to tell Helen how much I had enjoyed the shopping expedition, I could not. I wanted to, I pictured myself saying something – but it got lost on the road to 'Speech'.

My friendship with Helen did not really blossom until

after my return from England in the new year when I felt more sure of myself. But I was very grateful to Helen for offering friendship when she did and I missed her when she left for New Zealand a year later.

Four months after the stroke my handwriting grew quite bad again. I was trying to write faster. The mental effort and the physical task of writing did not tire me quite so much now. Whereas before I had written a line of two of very concrete observations now it seemed I was a little more expansive. But I still did not come out of the 'concrete' and into the 'abstract' for a while yet.

The concrete refers to our 'bread and butter' requirements. In a shop I might ask for some olives and salami at the delicatessen section which would be a concrete statement. At this stage I was fairly good at asking for things in shops as long as the staff did not try and engage me in conversation. I would have the word 'olives' ready in my mind before I went into the shop. If the shop assistant remarked that it was a 'nice day', it would not only make me forget my olives but throw me into a spin of stuttering from which I could not emerge without having to admit that I had been ill. What is not a concrete remark? If the shop assistant had said, 'Nice day' and I had replied, 'It would be a nice day for a walk' my remark would have been abstract. But whole areas of speculation and conjecture were being left out of my thoughts because I would have to resort to my imagination for such a fantasy. I could not readily do that. I could probably think of it laboriously (but still not connect it to 'Speech') in the next five minutes. But that was much too late.

Five months after the stroke it seemed that I had become a little quicker at putting my concrete thoughts - and even some abstract thoughts - on paper. I wrote what I thought was an impassioned letter to Ben, on hearing of some IRA atrocity committed against the Royal Marines. At that time Ben was keen on joining the Royal Marines. I tried hard to put him off when I heard about the IRA attempt. I was able to write four paragraphs (about half a side of A4 paper) compared with my usual effort of one or at most two paragraphs. I pictured it all in my mind, the fighting, the bombs and the burning buildings. I thought I was putting across the whole picture but really I was not. Nothing much came out on paper. I just thought it.

I started going to a Pentecostal church sometimes with Alan or Helen. I enjoyed the sermon immensely but I would not raise my hands in the air. I was brought up in the Church of England tradition and such flights from inhibition were not for me. I listened to the sermon which was usually on some practical aspect of life and the pastor was very entertaining. But when asked afterwards I could not discuss what he had been talking about. Later when my mind had pieced itself together again I was able to recall a little of these sermons. I think it is important for people with speech problems like mine to have the stimulation of as many talks as possible on different subjects. ABC radio national supplied much of what I needed.

A friend once thought about me when taking some books back to the library. In all good faith wanting to help, he took out a tape of a children's book and gave it to me to listen to. Did he think my poor speech reflected a poor mind? Of course he did and why shouldn't he? At least he was honest about it. At the time it just flung me back on my own resources. I had to think, 'What can I do to hasten my recovery?'. I knew it was all up to me. But it was that incident and a few other incidents that caused me to write this book on the reality of how I was feeling. If even my friends, who knew me well, could get the wrong idea of what was happening to me I could try to write about my condition and enlighten them that way.

CHAPTER TEN

The Mind Boggles

Chris, the speech pathologist for the Outward Bound Group took us on an excursion to the Maritime Museum in Fremantle in early November. There were six of us and we took the train. We all had trouble finding the right money for the fare. Ken and Yvonne laid their fingers down in order to count, it seemed a good idea so I tried it too and it helped.

We stopped for morning tea at a little cafe in Fremantle then we went on to the Maritime Museum. On the way Ken was talking to me as we crossed a railway line. He could not find the word for train. 'Toot toot', he said and we both started to laugh. Many times we did not realise we had made a mistake or used a 'near miss' word unless our audience looked at us enquiringly. On those occasions, if we had just said it we did remember. But when we had to look for a word we sometimes picked one close to it – and it was the best we could do. That was why some of us sounded so pedantic at times. 'Have you got the device for sealing the air out of bottles of wine?'[answer: a cork]. Or we might describe a 'repast' [meal] with 'cruciferous vegetables' [cabbage].

We wandered about in twos and threes in the museum. Wally made for the rebuilding of the *Batavia*. It was quite an achievement, sightseers could walk right round it on the decking. Ken tried to explain the working of an engine to me. I could tell he knew it backwards if he only had his speech. His 'Visualisation' was working overtime. He knew every move the engine would make but he could not get it into his 'Speech' compartment.

Ken was in the Navy and he told the group that when he first had his stroke, he tried to communicate in morse code to a naval friend who called to visit him – to no avail. Ken thought he had died and wanted to know for sure. Morse did not help because it works through the language centres and needs thought to generate it, in much the same way that speech does.

In *Seeing Voices*, Oliver Sacks (the author of *Awakenings*) states that sign language has grammar rules of its own and uses the same areas of the left brain as are used for speech – the area damaged in the type of stroke that Ken and I had. So even if I had known sign language and morse code before my stroke – and I did not – it would not have helped.

Dr Sacks says that gestures such as shrugging the shoulders, waving goodbye or brandishing a fist is retained in aphasia even though the ability to sign is not. From my own experience gesture became very useful for obtaining my basic needs. When right brain activity was mostly all that was left to me I could still make those gestures. For more complex ideas gesture was simply not adequate for the task. Because the complex ideas involved more thinking.

I could see how frustrated Ken must have been – we all were. Gesturing was very useful when what we needed was a glass of water or to turn to another television channel. But we needed something like a miracle for the abstract!

Despite our setbacks we enjoyed the outing thoroughly. The responsibility of looking after all of us must have been hard work for Chris at times. But these excursions helped to expand our experience and added to the learning process after our strokes. A little like the radio broadcasts, I felt they got our dendrites pulsing.

I keep stressing 'radio' and not 'television' because with my particular type of stroke I definitely did not need more visual stimulation. That is one area the stroke seemed not to have touched. Television supplies pictures and as an afterthought words. Television has little more than an eight hundred word vocabulary. I did not need that. Radio has only words with which to make pictures and that was more useful to me. The opposite might apply for other sorts of strokes.

One day Christine and I were on a shopping expedition and we were looking for a bookshop where they sold 'do-it-yourself' wills. I was concerned about the last one I had had professionally drawn up. I made it at a time when cardboard coffins were the latest trend. I wrote in the will that I wanted to be put into a cardboard coffin, cremated and my ashes scattered at sea. The typist had put that I was to be 'Cremated and my ashes put into a cardboard box'. With a stroke I had had a narrow escape and I fancied I could feel the 'Fates' tugging at my mortal thread. I was not going to leave things to chance and let bureaucracy botch anything up if I could help it.

At the bookshop I told Christine I would like to get a book about stroke to see how the person who wrote it had managed to cope. She said she knew of one written by a journalist called Ron Saw. Christine had read his newspaper column and said he was a very funny writer – 'That should cheer you up'. We found the book: *Stroke – And How I Survived It*.

I started reading it that night. It was a book that was warm and readable (even to someone with my disability). It was sensitive but I did not find it the least bit funny. I said to Christine when she telephoned, 'Perhaps having a stroke even knocks the humour out of someone like him'. Ron Saw's stroke was on the opposite side to mine; his damage was to the left-hand side if his body and the right-hand side of the brain. I wondered whether it had somehow affected his speech and writing as well, as in 'left-brain' damage.

I remember complaining bitterly about my lack of sense of humour to Christine and whoever else would listen to my moans. But I did not realise fully at that time in November that it was not that the book was not funny, I just failed to see the humour in it. In April 1990 nearly two years after the stroke I came across the book again and was idly thumbing through it. I thought, 'Hold on, this is funny – very funny!'. I immediately rang Christine and told her. I was dancing with glee.

After the stroke I noticed that my speech seemed to follow a path like the one we follow from early childhood – beginning with not being able to speak at all. It is a strange sensation losing one's speech in that way. I tended to regress and become very childlike then. As recovery slowly continued – and how slowly - I 'grew' up. A certain amount of timidity marks some parts of early childhood and sometimes a lack of confidence. It was not long then before I re-entered adolescence. Could it have been as bad as that the first time? There was not a day that went by when I did not embarrass myself utterly by something I had said.

The acute phase lasted for about one month then it gradually tempered itself so that I could usually control what I said. Suzanne was my speech pathologist at that time when the phase was at its peak. If only I had known then what I know now: that I became aware of a difficulty just before I had a brain click. A brain click usually seemed to follow awareness of the problem within about three to four weeks. I did not know this however and I resolved to stay silent rather than blurt something out.

One day I said to Suzanne, 'I feel uncomfortable, gauche like a fifteen year old'. Then I promptly proved it.

We were doing an exercise: Suzanne was miming an action and I had to guess what she was doing. She made swabbing movements over her arm. I thought, 'Blood?'.

Suzanne helped me out, 'Something light and soft' she said, 'applying medication'. I realise now it was meant to be 'cotton wool'.

'Vaginal cream!' I cried – not even 'Delfen' or 'contraceptive cream' which would have been slightly better. She and I relapsed into stunned silence from which Suzanne quickly recovered and changed the subject.

I was too miserable and embarrassed about the incident to tell her my mind was probably still 'one-tracking'. I had thought of 'blood' – it was just unfortunate that my next thought took me to 'menstruation' and then to 'contraceptive'. It was too hard to communicate and besides, at that time I only had fleeting insights into this brain of mine. I just could not grasp the concept in order to tell Suzanne. She must have gone away thinking, 'We've got a weird one here!'. I, for my part, took the trivial incident very much to heart like a teenager does. I later read that frontal lobe damage can result in the loss of some social inhibitions. Whatever the cause I was heartily glad to see the back of that phase.

It was during my one-month 'adolescence ' period that I saw Dr B for the second time since leaving the hospital. For him I picked the awful expression, 'It makes the mind boggle'. By the time I had repeated it three times, he repeated it amiably with me. There was nothing apparently I could do to stop myself from saying it. I was 'one-tracking' again – but whereas before it had been set off by a road sign or something someone said, now I was able to generate my own thoughts and repeat those again and again.

I think Suzanne really understood the problem. I told her that one of the worst things about the illness was not being able to read 'complicated' books something with 'meat' in it. 'I read them so slowly' I complained, 'they don't make sense any more'. She said, 'I sympathise with you the world of the imagination is just not open to you'.

I hated changes at that time. I had got used to Suzanne but she was a final year student and the time had come for her to move on. I was very sorry for myself. I burst into tears in front of her and her supervisor and walked sniffing from the room.

After the typing course I did not want to be left in the house with nothing to do. I signed on for a course in woodwork again at CYSS. I had done courses in woodwork before so it was not new to me. I felt that I had to keep my hands moving in all sorts of different ways. I knew that control of the human hand takes up a large part of the brain and thought that stimulating the hands would somehow flow on to stimulating the brain.

The woodwork shop was a fascinating place. Every so often a boy doing community work for the courts would appear among us. One of these laid some slabs for us; the woodworking shed was being expanded. Charlie, our teacher was very 'laid back'. He worked in a swirl of activity, there were people using the docking saw, one using the thicknesser (for smoothing wood), one even trying to paint toy trucks and engines amid the sawdust. Charlie was very good he growled when someone was not wearing protective glasses but remained serene apart from that. There was a woman there – the one trying to paint the toy trucks – who had been a fellow teacher at one of my previous schools. She had had a nervous breakdown.

I was very much at home doing woodwork. I made three chopping boards, one for CYSS to sell at a fête stall and the others for me. I had plans for them thinking they would make nice birthday presents.

I thought my right hand was normal by now. I soon found that it was not by any means. I could not use a chisel or a screwdriver. It was like working with two left hands. The chisel dug and gouged and I could not get the hang of the screwdriver at all. I discovered I had become incompetent with all things mechanical. It was not quite as bad or as noticeable at home. There I could not work the tin opener, I held it in a strange position so that even if I had got the right turning motion it still would not have opened the tin. To open my dishwasher which is portable and on wheels I kept grasping it by the rail I use to push it around, instead of the door handle. I generally had difficulty with anything that required the fingers to move in opposite ways, like eye shadow containers or clasps on purses.

I had been used to machinery before the stroke having worked in a laboratory and on farms. I loved gadgets but now it was different. The wood thicknesser with its razor-sharp blade made my blood run cold. I said nothing to Charlie, I took a deep breath and put my wood through. It worked! All that was required was a simple pushing movement. I tried not to let the uneasiness show on my face as I approached the band saw. It was easy just a matter of pushing again. Once I had mastered the brutes I did not find it a problem using them again and I really enjoyed the woodwork. I do not think Charlie ever knew quite what a liability I was.

I went to woodwork from November until it was time for my trip to England. It was very relaxing and like the typing course structured my day.

Like years and months, hours and days meant nothing to me. I suppose that was because I could not deal with figures successfully. When I arranged to do something on a particular day, for instance I might have arranged to go shopping with Yvonne – I would say, 'You'll have to tell me when that day is.' Yvonne would than count the days off for me on her fingers.

I was not as bad as I have heard some stroke patients can be. Some people cannot tell if it is night or day and get up and dress in the middle of the night and want their breakfast. I was spared that.

Imagine the fun I had when the itinerary arrived for my trip overseas. Naturally I tried to sort it out myself. I used to quite good at organising. If I took my time I thought this would present me with very few problems and none that I could not handle. I started to struggle with the times written as '1400 hr' and '0900 hr' changing them to two o'clock and so on. While I was doing this Rosemary came by. She helped me with some of it and then I made some coffee and we chatted – or rather, Rosemary chatted. My chatter was still very limited. If I disagreed with what was being said I usually came unstuck. I would wave my hands about and utter expletives. When I had Rosemary's attention out would come the first two or three words ...then it was lost again. I knew I did have a good point to make but I would finish lamely completely forgetting what I was going to say and, as likely as not, the conversation itself because I was upset. We did manage to establish the days on which I would be leaving various airports.

I used to be punctual but not any more. A hairdressing appointment in Perth at three in the afternoon would pose a problem for me. At this time I went by bus into the city, I did not trust myself to drive. The concentration would have been too much for me and I would have had very little energy left to find the hairdresser. The bus would take twenty minutes, the walk at each end of the bus would take fifteen minutes and the buses came every half hour. I tried to work it out in my head then on paper. When would I have to leave home? Even the thought of working it out made me shudder. I left home at twelve-thirty.

I realised that I was boring. I bored myself. The value of the typing and woodwork courses was that they kept me busy. I was not feeling bored while I was doing something practical but more to the point I was not being boring to other people either while I was doing it and I still had their company.

I was invited to Yvonne's daughter's twenty-first birthday party in November. I drove about a block in the dark to the hall where it was to be held. I was a bit unnerved when I reached the hall. Just driving in the dark and planning to be out late were enough to set me on edge. I had met many of the people who were to be at the party before but I did not know some of them very well. Some of Yvonne's friends were helping and I would have liked to help too. I cast around for something to do. One of the helpers pushed back some chairs. 'That's an idea' I thought. But it was all done. One of them stirred a mixture on the stove. That was another idea – but she tapped the spoon on the side of the saucepan and put it down, finished. I could not think of anything to do independently. Mike, seeing me standing there led me to a table and introduced me to the relatives. I sat there silent as stone once the introductions were over. This was a terrible ordeal having to try and make conversation to people. I need not have worried, they were quite aware of my condition and pretended not to notice. The effort involved in finding even one item of information that I could talk about was too much. So I spent the time watching the high-cholesterol biscuits and dips moving up and down the table. I could not have any.

I had perked up considerably and was quite enjoying myself when they put the strobe lights on to accompany the discotheque. All the other lights in the hall were put out and only the super-bright lights of the disco were shining. Silver lights, followed by red, green and yellow swept the hall at startling speeds. Of course I had encountered these things before my illness and they had not bothered me then. Why did I feel like bursting into tears now? Because that is exactly what I felt like doing. They had only been going two or three minutes and I wanted to howl! I knew that if I did not leave I would utterly disgrace myself and the last thing I wanted was to draw attention to myself. I bid the the aunts and uncles a hurried, 'Goodbye' with a smile even now faltering and rushed out. I left my car there and Mike drove me home.

I was reminded of a young man I heard about with epilepsy who fitted strobe lights above his bed and used to turn them on and induce a fit before he went to a disco. That way he could be sure that he would not have another fit for at least three or four hours and so he was safe to go dancing.

Away from the strobe lights I recovered from the experience. It was very thoughtful and kind of Yvonne and Mike to invite me; treating me as if I was a normal person was the best thing possible for me. It meant I could go on finding my own feet. At the time I did not like large gatherings of people: that in itself would be enough to make me agitated. As I came to realise later even people I knew well I could take better in ones and twos. I think this was because my attention was soon distracted by people and it was difficult enough to concentrate when there were just a few people let alone at a party. It was as if my attention wandered equally between any groups that were within hearing range. It was all right when I was not speaking. I would pick up conversations that went like, 'I see a cure's been found for dog tick fever...', 'Wouldn't you think that Ann would be...', 'And I said, "Go for it" and he did...'. I would begin my own sentence with whatever appealed to me most: 'Go for it...I'd like another champagne, dog tick'.

Yes, parties can be miserable events for those of us who have had stokes. I would probably have coped better had I not been on my own. I began to feel sorry for myself, not having an understanding husband to take care of me – but I had to be careful of that sort of negative thinking.

One sunny day when it was not too hot I took my bag of clubs down to the golf course. I was prepared to play by myself as it was the first time I had played since my illness. I did not want to hold anyone up. I envisaged myself going down the fairway in a series of small chip shots – or worse, going down the rough in a series of even smaller chip shots. But the course was crowded and the professional asked me to play with another woman golfer. Brenda really looked the part. She even had a pencil to mark our cards (nobody ever has a pencil). She was very professional. I thought, 'Oh well, we'll be held up by the foursome in front. She won't bother about me.'. Brenda was certainly a good player but my tee shot was quite good too. I heaved a sigh of relief and settled down to enjoy the game. It was a perfect Perth day, warm with a slight breeze. The walk alone did me good.

Although my fairway shots were quite good and I did not slice or pull unduly, my putting was atrocious. It had never been as bad as this. I had no idea of the amount of back-swing to use, or how hard to hit the ball or about direction. I was glad it was only on the green that I was quite so awful.

I had taken a card for nine holes. I got very tired towards the end of the nine and my game deteriorated. For one reason or another I have not played since but it is good to know that I can.

Around this time I noticed I had begun to dress with more care. I no longer went down to the local shops without make-up and wearing thongs and jeans. This came about directly because of my poor speech. I had come to realise that quite a few people I met when I went out were a bit hostile to me. This was not my imagination; it was real. I did not tell the girl at a busy checkout that I had had a stroke but nevertheless she could see that I was different. She may have noticed me fumbling in my purse and coming out with the wrong change. She may have been disconcerted by my 'head down' approach and refusal to smile. She may have been convinced that I was drunk. Whatever the reason it was not pleasant to be treated as if I was odd. I could not bite back with a barbed comment. Even if I had been lucky enough to think of one in time – I could not have delivered it. It made me feel vulnerable. So to compensate I dressed as well as I could when I appeared in public.

Normally of course there is no need to 'bite back'. People just do not look at you in an appraising way when you are acting the way everybody else acts. But if you act differently people treat you differently and in my case I could not say anything about it. No wonder I dressed with care. And it worked. I could tell people were thinking twice before giving me a hard stare.

The lack of speech ate right into my dealings with the outside world. It made me vulnerable, timid, defensive and shy. I hated being like that. I used to have opinions and laugh and tell stories.

CHAPTER ELEVEN

Left Luggage

I was really looking forward to my trip to England which was in December 1988 (five months after the stroke). I had been able to put my departure date back two weeks because I was no longer tied to school holidays. It was cheaper that way. So I planned to stay for one night in Singapore on the way out and three nights on the way back with the money I had saved on the fare. The three nights on the return journey turned out to be a disaster. I panicked and ended up flying home after only one night.

I left Sunil (whom I had met at the typing course) in charge of my house. I would not have bothered asking someone to house-sit if I had not been worried about my cat. My neighbours had always minded the house for me when I was away for short periods but I thought Hiraeth had been insecure for too long and that another spell with me away from the house might be too much for him. He might wander off. I showed Sunil how to lift Hiraeth up onto the bench for his supper. Hiraeth liked to be lifted up. Sometimes he would jump up himself to see what I had given him and then jump off again and wait to be lifted up.

Michael and Lynette looked after Maggie. They have a house in the country and a corgi of their own called Ferdie. Maggie would be well taken care of there. Not only that they had a swimming pool and Maggie adored swimming. It would be just the thing to help heal her broken leg.

All I had left to do was the packing. I was reminded of the the time about three months before the stroke when Yvonne and I were going for a weekend camping trip. Then I had been so slow – painfully slow. Usually Ben packed the van for me. But even when I did it myself it would usually take only about an hour. That time just before the stroke it had taken me over four hours.

Packing for the holiday in England was just as bad. I just could not get organised and the experience was maddening. I had all the clothes that I wanted to take with me strewn across the dining room table. There were far too many. The sensible person at this stage begins to cull some. But that would have involved me in mathematics: how many days was I staying? It was too hard. I washed and ironed some more and piled those up too. I gratefully left the mounting heap when Christine suggested we go into town and finish off the odds and ends there like the airport tax and buying an Akubra hat as a present for Ben.

Christine's help was very welcome. After explaining to her

what I wanted to do and where I wanted to go I felt as if a load had been lifted off my shoulders. Left to myself I would probably have weaved my way across town concentrating too hard and getting too tired, visiting the bank, the post office and the stores in no logical order. Christine sorted all that out for me.

It strikes me now that my problem was making a decision. When I look back on the camping trip, the packing or that trip round town they were fraught with decisions. Deciding what to do next remained incomprehensible to me for a long time.

I worked out what to pack eventually. But it took a week instead of hours to do. I did not take anything foolish nor did I forget anything important. My passport, ticket and traveller's cheques (I had to think about traveller's cheques and arrange them myself) were all ready. I was very proud of myself.

I was excited to be going at last. Alan, Christine and Rosemary saw me off at the airport. As far as I knew everything I needed was packed, the dog and cat were in good hands and Ben would be meeting me at Heathrow. All that remained for me to do was to get myself from Perth to London.

I had ordered low-cholesterol meals on the plane. A lot of people when I told them this, said, 'They'll just give you vegetarian meals – without cream'. They did not. The low-cholesterol food on QANTAS (at that time) was magnificent. It even included beautifully cooked steak instead of the usual steamed fish, which they tend to resort to monotonously on some of the other airlines. It was delicious – and with no visible fat on it at all. The beauty of it was that even though I had a glass of wine with my meals I had no jet-lag at all. Although a sample of one is nothing to go by, I for one am going to eat low-cholesterol meals on aeroplanes from now on.

All was going well until I reached Singapore where I was to

have the one-day stopover. I should have been better prepared. I should have booked into a hotel as near the airport as possible, ordered a meal by room service, had a shower and gone to bed. I did none of those things.

Oh, the foolishness of my thinking. Some of my friends wanted me to have a 'good time'. Should they have known better? Maybe not; after all they were lulled into thinking I must have been well on the road to recovery to even contemplate a trip like this. And I had none of the outward signs, like paralysis, that would perhaps have reminded them of the seriousness of my illness. I now know that I was not fit to go sightseeing after the near shave I had had – taking a holiday in England, yes; sightseeing, no. But at the time I thought I was all right.

Tom had given me a list of places to see in Singapore. He had included the Botanic Gardens, a tour of the harbour and the colourful shopping arcade Change Alley. To my dismay it was raining in Singapore which I had not expected and I was told the monsoons would last until January when I was to make my return journey.

I think there is nothing so dejected as a basically hot country when it is raining. There are not many people about but those who are wear skimpy shirts and dresses because it is still quite warm in spite of the rain. Swimming pools are under wraps and management takes the opportunity to perform maintenance while no one is swimming, giving them a desolate air. Nobody wears the good solid 'macs' of the European countries or carries umbrellas. The buildings look drab, many of them naked concrete relieved by marble and glass. The light in the Southern Hemisphere is full of orange, yellow and red and it does not take kindly to the look of rain. As a consequence everything looks washed out and dull because rain is so different from sunshine: soft and moody as rain is, in my opinion it needs the violet, blue the lemon of the northern hemisphere to make it look its best.

The hotel where I was staying was about ten kilometres from the airport and I was taken there by a tour operator in a small bus. The tour operators stand outside the customs gates waving placards with names on them – so I managed to find the right bus to the hotel.

I was feeling distinctly odd by the time I arrived at the hotel. I was very tired and I wondered how I was going to manage at the hotel desk. They did not ask me much at the desk, much to my relief and gave me a key to a room on the twelfth floor. Bearing in mind I was still at the stage where an idea, once put into my head tended to stay there. It was not surprising that I had a shower and went downstairs to find something to eat because I had intended to do that from the start. This was very silly.

I looked at the menu for the exclusive restaurant. That was too expensive. I really only wanted a sandwich. I knew there was a coffee shop somewhere. While I was looking for that I happened across a bar and went in.

If I were to write a list of 'don't do's' for people recovering from a stroke one of them would be: 'Don't drink when you feel tired'. I had a gin and tonic – and then another one because it was 'Happy Hour'. The band and the alcohol and the lack of food in my stomach all conspired to make me weepy. One of the band winked at me in a friendly way. I just got out of the bar in time before the tears started to trickle down my face. I was exhausted.

Strangely although I was hungry and tired when I got back in my room it still did not occur to me to eat. I might have thought to look in the hotel guide for room service but I did not. It is quite peculiar when you cannot change your mind when the circumstances warrant it. In the end I went to bed without having anything to eat.

I went down to breakfast the next morning feeling a lot better. One of the people whom I had seen on the bus came in after me and we had breakfast together. She had planned to go on a shopping tour and invited me to go with her. I did not feel too inhibited about my speech. I was quite able to make unspectacular comments like, 'Isn't that nice' or 'Lovely'. I enjoyed myself and we ended up at the Raffles Centre for coffee and then returned to the hotel by taxi.

But if I had not been invited on that shopping trip I would have spent a lamentable day clinging to the hotel and waiting for the plane to go. It occurred to me that I really could not enjoy myself without speech. I only had to have one misunderstanding with a bus driver or a waiter and whatever confidence I had mustered would evaporate. And in fact on the return journey to Perth I did not meet anyone going to the same hotel and I spent the time alone. What was the problem? I could have taken a trip in a tourist bus after all. But that was too hard. And I still had the problem of time. I could not tell if a given tour would be finished in time for me to get to the airport to catch my plane.

When it was time to be taken back to the airport I searched and re-searched my room for anything I might have left behind. That Shenton Park nurse had done a brilliant job.

Having four hours to kill at the airport before the plane took off I piled my suitcases onto an airport trolley and was ambling around with that when I came across the 'left luggage' office. I could see people queuing up and depositing their bags. I thought crazily to myself, 'That's a good idea'. So why was I the only person in the airport with their baggage still on a trolley? It was a terrible nuisance. I could not take the baggage upstairs to sit on the more comfortable chairs. I had to drag it with me when I went looking for postcards – to say nothing of having to look after it when I had one of my endless cups of coffee. And where was I to put it when, one coffee too many I had to visit the toilet? I do not know why I did not take advantage of the 'left luggage' office. Maybe it was a feeling of not knowing when to collect my cases again. But it was more likely that I did not visualise it as relating to me.

The trip was uneventful until I disembarked at Heathrow and Ben was not there to meet me.

I sat and waited. Perhaps there was some delay as he was catching the train to Heathrow from Bristol. The thought consoled me for a little while. I eventually thought back to the evening he had telephoned me to find out my flight number. Of course I had given him the wrong time! After all my translating of the twenty-four hour clock times I had given him the wrong one. He did not know of my difficulty with numbers. I found out later that Ben had rung the airport to check on the time but by then when he had realised my mistake, I was on a local flight to Heathrow from Stockholm. He could not possibly make it in time. (Many people did not have mobile telephones then).

I waited at the airport from ten in the morning until two in the afternoon by which time I had had more than enough. I lugged my suitcases on a trolley over to the bus station and enquired about buses to Weston-Super-Mare in the South West of England where my mother lives. I had just missed a bus. The next was at five in the evening. By this time I was heartily wishing I had not come at all, as I went out to where I had precariously left my bags without supervision. Such is the way of some modern architectural thinking: there was a steep step down at the entrance to the enquiries office so that travellers could not wheel their baggage in.

I was just about to leave the office when it occurred to me to ask about buses going to Bristol instead as there were other buses from Bristol to Weston-Super-Mare every half hour. 'There is one to Bristol leaving from London every hour' the girl said stifling a yawn. Why hadn't she said so in the first place? I was furious, with myself for not thinking of it before and with her for not telling me. Besides I was so tired. It had cost me dearly that foray in the enquiries office in used up concentration.

When I joined the queue I had been awake so long that I had become light-headed. The bus roared in and the driver, an athletic-looking young man jumped to the ground and undid the lock to the baggage compartment. Then he stood there flirting with the female crew member who had crawled untidily from the bus and was also standing there twitching her skirt. Meanwhile old ladies who presumably were used to the system struggled, pushed and wriggled their cases into the baggage compartment. Our hero would only help when some old lady threatened to expire and present him with the inconvenience of having to write a report on the incident. Of course I would have to do likewise but for a dear old man who had helped his wife with her baggage and then insisted on helping me with mine. The England I had arrived in had certainly changed.

It was a double-decker bus so having stowed my luggage in the compartment underneath I went upstairs. The upper level was full of the strangest-looking people: young, sprawled about the seats with vacant faces, untidy, hair dishevelled. I began to get nervous as a youth was looking fixedly at my purchases in a bag marked 'Changi Airport'. I decided to go downstairs. Someone told me conspiratorially that 'drug addicts' ride around on the top deck of buses.

It was dark by the time we pulled into Bristol bus station.

The bus stopped five metres from the kerb and began to pant and rev with impatience. I was ready for it this time and I asked the new male driver to help me carry my baggage to the kerb. He gave me a look of utter disbelief making me repeat my request. I persisted and to my amazement he complied.

By this time I had had time to think about 'left luggage'. In Bristol bus station there were no baggage carts. I had to swing a piece of luggage in front of me as far as I could drag the two other pieces up to it, then begin again. I thought of offering the teenage girls and boys who were sitting around on newspapers a pound to move my luggage but thought better of it. So I swung, dragged, swung, dragged until I came at last to the 'left luggage' office. I was able to leave the largest bag there to be collected in the morning.

I changed buses. It was dark by now although it was still only five o'clock. The bus went the 'country way' to Weston-Super-Mare and I began to regain my flagging spirits. I was one of only five people on the bus and I enjoyed the tiny, high-banked country lanes, where cars would have to back up to let the bus through. There were villages with duck ponds and ancient pubs, the residents tucked up warmly against the cold night, windows glowing. The bus driver found me a telephone and I tried to call home without success. Ben was not there.

The driver dropped me in town where I could catch another bus to my mother's house. And then my journey would be at an end. It seemed to me that I had been travelling forever. It puzzled me that there were no buses with the familiar 'Bristol Omnibus' on the side. I was told that the company had been privatised. Now, there were lots of buses some of them double-decker and some of them eight-seater minibuses. There are a lot of pensioners living in Weston-Super-Mare and these little buses made it possible for them to get out of their houses.

Being small the minibuses did not have to stay on the main roads but could go in and out of the suburbs where they were really needed. My driver dropped me right outside the house. My faith in the English was returning.

The house was locked and in darkness there was a note from Ben that he had left the key at a neighbour's house in case he missed me while he went to Heathrow.

After a pleasant time renewing my acquaintance with the neighbours, Babs and Ron, Ron saw me home. We had just got in when in walked my lovely, grown-up son. If there is any consolation for having your son living in another country for two years it is that you really notice the changes in him. I was so proud of him: tall, slim and very mature. He had been in training and the dedication of that alone would have made a difference.

Looking back now at the entries in my diary I am surprised my friends let me go to England at all. The best word I can think of for my condition at that time is 'distorted' – and that puts it mildly! When I asked my friends about it later they said, 'We couldn't stop you'.

I was blithely unaware of course of my own incompetence. One of the few mercies of my stroke was that I did not know how bad I was.

I had quickly become accustomed to life in my own home in Perth. All I had to deal with there were the occasional telephone calls from people I did not know, other calls being from friends who knew about my condition. The local store stocked most of my requirements and they knew about the stroke too. At home I could concentrate on my speech alone. When concentration was too much for me no one was there to take note of the frequent rests I had to take. But it was a very different thing taking a holiday away from everything that had become familiar to me.

I coped for six weeks in a half-world of unreality. Ben was my anchor. We bought a small, decrepit car and walked every day in the lovely countryside of the Mendip Hills. And then Ben would go for a twenty kilometre run. Walking was no exercise he told me. It was quite enough for me. I began to feel fit and my speech improved. Quite hard exercise does improve the speech I found and I noticed when I took up swimming later that my speech improved noticeably again.

Among the examples of my distortion were temper tantrums – yes, temper tantrums! In public. Oh, that the earth could swallow me up. Ben's girlfriend and her mother watched me in fascinated horror while I childishly refused to eat the food put in front of me in a charming English pub.

Another example was that I was really unaware of money. For instance if I had been thinking properly I would have taken a taxi and checked into a hotel to wait for Ben at Heathrow instead of panicking. I did not seem to realise that the money I had would make my life easier. It may have been my unawareness of money that made me lug my bags round Changi instead of leaving them in the 'left luggage' office. Ben loves books and we were looking around the bookshop at Heathrow before I flew back to Australia. It never occurred to me to give him my excess English currency to buy some.

But there was one thing I did do right. Ben and I went to the Peak District (in Staffordshire) to a farm where I had spent half of my childhood. The people there were a second family to me and I had grown up with their children.

Ben and I went on journeys of complete nostalgia – for me. We walked down the Manifold Valley, visited the old farm at Swainsley, went to Leek on market day and had Guinness at the Black Lion. It was on this visit, on the 10th of January 1989 that I became aware of brain clicks for the first time. Suddenly the world seemed more expansive, larger, and I felt more in tune with it. My speech and fluency improved and I felt ready to move on.

Seeing my mother and Ben again and seeing the places that I grew up in made me feel that I was returning to my roots. I am glad nobody persuaded me not to go even though I must have missed half of it through lack of awareness.

CHAPTER TWELVE

Too Slow

When I arrived back in Perth in January 1989 the temperature was 43° Celsius. Alan met me at the airport and took me home.

Up until then I had had things to occupy me like the thought of my trip back home. I had been still very much an invalid so getting better was the main thing on my mind. But now what?

I soon grew bored and very depressed. The drama was over. Friends had got used to not telephoning me while I was away. Sometimes I went two or three days without a call. I could have telephoned them but I asked myself, 'Who wants to hear from a person who has very little to say, no imagination and stutters?'.

My general practitioner put me on antidepressants again.

Was I ready for a job of some sort? Somewhere I did not have to count – or answer the telephone?

In early February I telephoned two or three hospitals to ask about the availability of ward assistants' jobs. I would be able to count out a few sheets I felt. I wrote down a small set speech to read out when somebody answered the telephone. Luckily they did not want to talk to me they just took down my name.

This exercise was not satisfactory: I wanted something to happen. The head speech pathologist at Bentley Hospital, Melita Brown suggested I make an appointment to see the Commonwealth Rehabilitation Service. I took Rosemary along for moral support and in case I missed anything important. They were very helpful and the gist of their message was: 'We'll help you get back in the workforce by putting you in a job (for instance a library assistant) and allowing the library to pay you just enough so that your pension is not interfered with'. At the same time there would be ongoing courses in assertiveness, relaxation and so on. I was all ready to do that when South Perth Community Hospital rang and invited me for an interview for a full-time job as a kitchen assistant.

I was interviewed by Sister Lynne Tidy who told me that subject to the approval of Ms Colleen McIntosh (the Director of Nursing) I could have the job. Ms McIntosh raised no objection and I was to start the next day the 7th of February 1989. My duties included serving meals on trays to patients, making salads and sandwiches, washing up and generally helping in the kitchen.

I began by having three days of induction into the system. By morning tea I was exhausted but there was the whole of the day to get through yet. I thought I would never do it. What would it be like when I started the real work? I dragged myself somehow through the rest of the day, went home and without even a cup of tea went straight to bed.

On the second day about morning tea time my eyelid began to twitch again. In a burst of fury I said to the eyelid, 'Do what you like – I'm not stopping just because of you' and it stopped. I was so surprised, I decided I should start talking to all my symptoms like that.

The kitchen seemed mercifully dark at first. I could not see much. While I was there Ms McIntosh had the floors painted cream but that did not make any difference to my perception of the kitchen as a dark place. It became gradually lighter over about a year, a pleasant place to work in, sunlight through the windows and plenty of fresh air.

Some time later I heard a radio broadcast of William Styron (who wrote *Sophie's Choice*) talking about his book *Darkness Visible*. He said that when depression is upon us we see the world as a dark place. I was not aware of being depressed at that time; on the contrary I was ecstatic to have the job and excited about it. But perhaps the world on occasion seems dark when we are under extreme duress; when we do not have time to look at it; when we are too concerned with looking internally.

My colleagues in the kitchen were Rod, the catering supervisor. Sandra and Peter the full-time cooks and Winnie the relief cook. I peered at them blankly out of my darkness and hurriedly withdrew. I did not even try to remember the names of the 'girls' with whom I would be working.

My duties should not have been too difficult. But I had not bargained for my appalling slowness.

I seemed to have no forward thinking ability even when I had been there for a while. When I had finished a job like wrapping the cutlery in a serviette I would just stand there. In a busy kitchen I knew there was something else to do. But what?

I racked my brain and still could not think. Somebody would say 'You could put the bags in the teapots' and off I would go again with all the speed and direction of a demented jellyfish, tentacles in a twist, flailing nowhere, until I would get to the 'Now what?' stage again. 'You could put the teapots away, now' – and so it went on. I watched what the other 'girls' did and followed them – *exactly!* - many is the time when I grabbed a cloth and witlessly followed along behind someone, doing the same thing, until they turned and snarled at me, 'I've already done that – and that - and that.' And I was not really aware I was quite so slow.

For about three months they carried me. Sandra, Peter and Rod must have wondered what they had taken on. They were patient with me and covered with a laugh many things that must have driven them to distraction.

I was generally sent on the afternoon tea round, one of two assistants. On our trolley were trays that we were to load with a little jug of milk, a teapot and a jug, which we filled from the urn on the trolley, a cup and a plate for some delicious cake or other (I soon put on four kilogrammes working there, in spite on the low-cholesterol diet I tried to maintain). I approached the task with a randomness that a statistician would have envied. I would start one tray with the plate; another with the jugs; another still with the packets of sugar, forgetting about the cup. Finally when my partner had finished the whole corridor I would emerge from a patient's room to find the trolley gone.

I did not like changes. When I first started the teabag tin was kept on the side directly under 'Matron's Tray'. It was later moved to the other side beside the cutlery. I could not accept the change. I worried about it and kept putting it back in its 'right place'. It was just as useful one side as the other.

It was not only the teabag tin that I worried about. I did

not like taking morning tea to one side of the ward when I had become accustomed to taking it to the other side first. We took on quite a few new staff just after I arrived and it took me weeks to adjust to that.

The worst thing of all in those first few weeks was having to say 'Good Morning' – especially to Peter. He insisted that I use his name as well: 'Good Morning, Peter'. I sweated over practising 'Good Morning, Peter' when I knew he would be there. I would take a deep breath by the kitchen door and go in. I did not have long to wait; Peter's continually revolving eye on the 'workings' of his kitchen usually caught me coming in the door. 'Good Morning, Jenny' he would say.

If I had practised enough I could say 'Good morning... Peter' my voice fading with the effort. But if by any chance I was distracted, I was finished. If my eye happened to fall on Sue, I could not remember the 'Peter'. So I would say 'Good morning...'. And Peter would wait for me. He would stop what he was doing momentarily, fix me with a baleful stare and say, 'Spit it out!'. I do not know what the speech pathologists would have made of that – but it seemed to work!

Peter was often exasperated with me. Serving out the meals I sometimes put the meals in the wrong hotbox. He burst out in that histrionic way he has and roared, 'I'm going to write a book too, called: "I had to work with her."

Peter's bark was worse than his bite. He was really very kind and patient and so were Rod and Sandra.

I lived in daily fear of losing my job. I knew that I annoyed the girls I worked with because of my slowness. I could not blame them, sometimes when we were busy and I was on we did not finish until seven o'clock at night and the shift ended at six-thirty. One by one they applied to be put on the wards.

Peter egged on by grumbles from the girls I think applied

to Ms McIntosh to have me removed from the kitchen to 'Flowers and Laundry' where I could go at my own pace. I stuck it out for one day. The loneliness got to me most, that and the fact that I was reminded of my own time in hospital. I did the flowers in two rooms with tears overflowing. Finally I could stand it no longer. I rushed to Ms McIntosh's office still in tears and asked her to put me back in the kitchen.

'I'm back in the kitchen...Peter.'

Peter quickly pulled himself together. 'Oh! ...well...that's good.'

In the morning I went to Ms McIntosh and apologised for the outburst of tears.

Another thing I was worried about was the fact that I never smiled. And even if I could have talked, I rarely did for fear that I would lose what little concentration I had. I mentioned it to Sandra one day. Of course the tears started again – there was nothing I could do to stop the tears! I said, 'I'm sorry I never l...l...look very happ...y. It's because I have to concentrate so hard.' Sandra was very sweet and told me not to worry and that if I felt I needed to I could sit and rest for a while. I felt better having talked to her about it – and I never needed the rest.

I avoided the telephone as much as possible but the day came when I was standing right beside it when it rang. I had been in the kitchen then for about three weeks. Everyone was studiously looking the other way as they no doubt do in kitchens all over the world – whoever answered the telephone also carried out the request, whatever it was – and I was left with it. It was a nursing sister about to order her lunch. Her no-nonsense tones swam down the telephone at me, 'I want the pork medallions in orange sauce, a side salad and apricot crumble, jelly and icecream, please.' Puzzled she said, 'Are you there? Oh, good' and rang off. But she was dealing with me, poor thing who considered it an achievement just to have lifted the telephone at all. I was utterly baffled. The message had to be put in the book on the counter. It was one thing to remember what she had said (and I did not), another thing again to write it down. My writing was a jumble of capital letters interspersed with small letters and liable to fluctuating size differences – and I was upset which made it worse. I put it in the 'too hard' basket and promptly forgot all about it – until lunchtime when the sister came looking for her lunch. Suddenly the incident returned to me.

Docile to the point of imbecility I did not like to upset anybody. This was my 'timid' phase. One of the women who was leaving offered me a uniform. It was a size 16 (I take a size 12) and also it was very long. I knew I would have to give explanations if I was not going to take it, so I paid the $10 she was asking. I appeared in this monster of a uniform the next day. Towards the end of the day it began to dawn on me how ridiculous I looked and I was determined not to wear it again, no matter how many people I upset. The same person had a pair of enormous shoes that she said she would bring in the next day. By that time I was ready with an answer: 'No!'.

Working in a kitchen it is surprising just how much one needs to have an understanding of time and numbers.

Everything in a kitchen needed to be done at a set time. The morning tea trolley had to leave the kitchen at 10.30 am. But worse it had to be set up at 10.25 am. Time was meaningless to me (it did not get much better until thirteen months after my stroke). I had no trouble being able to see the clock or where the hands or the numbers were. But try as I might time itself did not make any sense. At 10.15 am I could not work out that I had ten minutes to go before we had to set up the trolley. I tried to count the minutes on the clock, visualise the

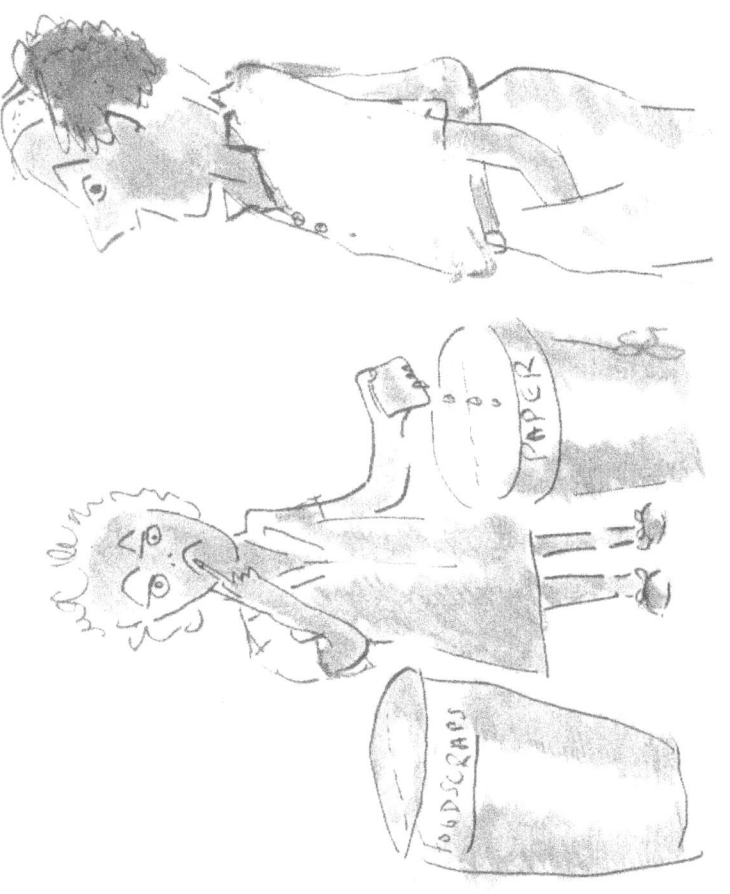

'If I were you, I'd put it in 'food scraps'.

spaces between them and think what that meant in time. But I could not count either. Giving up the unequal struggle, I just watched the other girls and followed them.

We made a list early in the morning of the things that we had to prepare in advance: the salads and sandwiches and other bits and pieces. I counted on the list; six salads then added two more for those people who changed their minds about having a hot lunch, three for staff...and somehow I must have doubled it: I made twenty-six salads! There were plates of salad in the cool-room, in the fridge, everywhere. And I had used up most of the plates.

More a matter of visualising were the sandwiches. We had shredded lettuce, grated carrot, sliced meat and chutney and other things all ready to use. I had to count a few times that I had enough slices of bread laid out on my board – one round per patient. Then I could not think what to put in them. The curried egg looked nice. So did the ham...what about cheese? I could not make decisions at all.

This applied to a lot of things. I asked Rod once if I should put used teabags in the 'Paper' waste or 'Food Scraps' waste. I could not make the decision myself. 'That's a good question' he said. 'Hmm...they've got paper on them and food inside.' And without the flicker of a grin he told me, 'I would personally put them in 'Food Scraps'.

I was slow partly because of these terrible decisions and partly because I could not think of the next thing to do.

Another problem was the concentration needed for every little thing about my work. I could not take anything for granted.

Teapots were my bête noire. As they came out of the dishwasher I could not at first separate them from the water jugs despite the fact that they were quite different. I had to resort to visualisation to sort them into categories. That worked but it took a lot of energy and concentration. Consequently I dragged myself to work each day feeling ever more tired. Finally I told myself, 'You have GOT to do this; if necessary you'll have to go to bed as soon as you get home from work and everything else will have to wait'. No wonder I never smiled.

People who have had a stroke like mine will probably be interested in when I considered that I started to recover. It seems to me that my recovery began the 'wrong' way. I first noticed it in July 1989 a year after the stroke when I called my co-worker Shirley a bitch.

There were always two of us on the early morning shift which began at 6.00 am. We divided the jobs into 'washing up' and 'setting the trays'. I had elected to do 'washing up' when I found the dishwasher was out of order. This meant I would have to wash up by hand and it would take me twice as long.

I wanted to say to Shirley, 'Let's do half and half: I'll help you with the trays and you help me with the washing up'. Needless to say it did not come out of my mouth like that. Waving at the pile of dirty dishes and thoroughly worked up already I spluttered, 'Those...those...that...all those dishes...we'll have to do half each'. I finished on a gasp.

Shirley whose own English was not the best (it was her second language) and who was already busy with the trays said vaguely, 'Yes. You agreed to do that job.'

Whenever I wanted to say something I had to blurt it out in short bits otherwise I would lose my concentration and forget what I was saying. I tried again extremely agitated by now. Shirley meanwhile had not looked around to see what all the fuss was about. 'Look you...you've ...we must...do it half and half" I cried.

I could not make her understand. She just went on putting

the cutlery on the trays. The hospital was full and we were at our busiest. Poor Shirley she was probably thinking she would be doing my job (as well as her own) in any case – so what was new? Again she refused shaking her head – probably in bewilderment. So I called her a bitch. I got her attention.

I was surprised by the word myself. I was definitely over-reacting but with troubled speech there are not many alternatives. It was the word I thought of first and because that word took up residence in the speech part on my brain it would have taken a complete change of subject to shift it. But I regretted it instantly. Shirley had been particularly nice to me when I first arrived taking me under her wing and pointing out things that needed to be done so I would not get the team's back up quite so much. Fortunately we can laugh about the incident now.

But I could not explain that to the Deputy Director of Nursing when Shirley took the story to her in tears.

On the credit side I was not letting people walk all over me quite so much. But still it is a pity I picked Shirley to try my wings out on.

This shift in my behaviour away from the 'timid' phase was to such an extent that I became downright intolerant. It was different from the 'temper tantrums' I described earlier. As I started to talk more I became more frustrated with myself and my lack of speech and I snapped at those around me. Invariably it was over silly little things. It seemed as if my inhibitions did not come back to the same speed as my speech. I was intolerant with new people who put things in the wrong places. I even knew that I was being unreasonable but that did not stop me. I shouted at one of the girls (who happened to leave soon after). She wanted the soup in her 'hot box' (the portable receptacle from which hot meals were served) instead of in mine. It was the first time I had raised my voice: I stuttered and coughed and went red in the face but I was proud of myself for defending the meals.

My frustration made me irritable and bad-tempered at home as well. Christine was making some curtains for Ben's room. I thought I knew better than her how to match up the pattern but of course I did not. Christine is a professional dressmaker. But still I hovered over the curtains supervising.

Someone picked up a square I was knitting for a blanket appeal and I was annoyed. Reaction first; think later, became the order of the day.

The girls whom I worked with were nice to me and they were tolerant as well. We had our tea breaks in the canteen and previously I had sat almost silently through these. Quite suddenly it seemed I was joining in the conversation and making remarks from time to time – and occasionally I would make a brief joke! I felt as if I was accepted by the girls more now than before: when I did not say much it was hard for people to get to know me. My co-worker Lorraine said I had more of a sense of humour. I felt I had arrived!

Through going to work I was able to pace myself every day and I noticed changes in my ability to do things. For instance we rolled the cutlery in serviettes every day and suddenly after twelve months I found it much easier to do. The job itself did wonders for my recovery. One day in October 1989 I found myself singing as I worked. I had tried to sing before but with no success: the 'tune' had come out as a monotone and without words. The first songs to come back were the first I had learnt: 'Sing a Song of Sixpence' followed by a selection from 'early musicals'. At last my love of music was coming back.

CHAPTER THIRTEEN

Tin Roofs and Mezzanine Floors

If one loses several levels of one's accumulation of ideas (by stroke or accident) then several years of life experience are also lost. I felt as if I were going through childhood all over again in some ways. I can see the reason for that feeling now. One goes through life growing more dendrites in the brain with every year that passes as more things are experienced. With my stroke I believe I regressed back to childhood (in some parts of my mind) and all that I had learned – speech, understanding and many skills – was lost. It was crushing to realise I had lost everything I had learned before – and now I had to relearn it.

I am sure though that the brain clicks I experienced somehow helped me to get back to normality more quickly than if I had to grow most of the dendrites from first principles (as a very young child has to do). That would be a lifetime's job starting all over again. It seems to come back much more quickly with the brain clicks: the neuron networks seem to be waiting for the recovery.

With a brain click I became suddenly aware of more things – the 'big picture' – and my level of understanding went up. It was so meaningful that things I had been thinking before the brain click happened seemed illogical to me now.

All my brain clicks seemed to happen at night – and they did not occur at regular intervals. I did not have to have a brain click in order to improve. I got better, very gradually all the time. However, the brain clicks were dramatic breakthroughs. When I went to bed one night at one stage of recovery and woke up the next morning at another; able to speak better and understand more and with everything falling better into place.

On the 7th of April 1989 for example I became a lot more organised, more chatty as well. I told Sandra about the farm in Staffordshire where my friends lived. This was unheard of for me at the time. I actually formed two sentences and I initiated the topic as well. At the same time I noticed that I was not so tired. This I put down to not having to concentrate on things so much. A brain click that occurred on the 5th of May 1989 was even more dramatic. Along with the better speech it produced I was able to formulate ideas. Previously I had had no sense of repartee I began to use a little now. People noticed.

With a brain click on the 25th of August 1990 I told a joke. I tried it on Peter. Leaning on the hot box for moral support, Peter sighed dramatically and looked at his watch. 'I suppose I've got a couple of hours to spend', he grumbled. 'Let's have it.' I told my joke word perfectly and without stumbling. Peter looked at me and said, 'Jenn, I'm proud of you.' It was

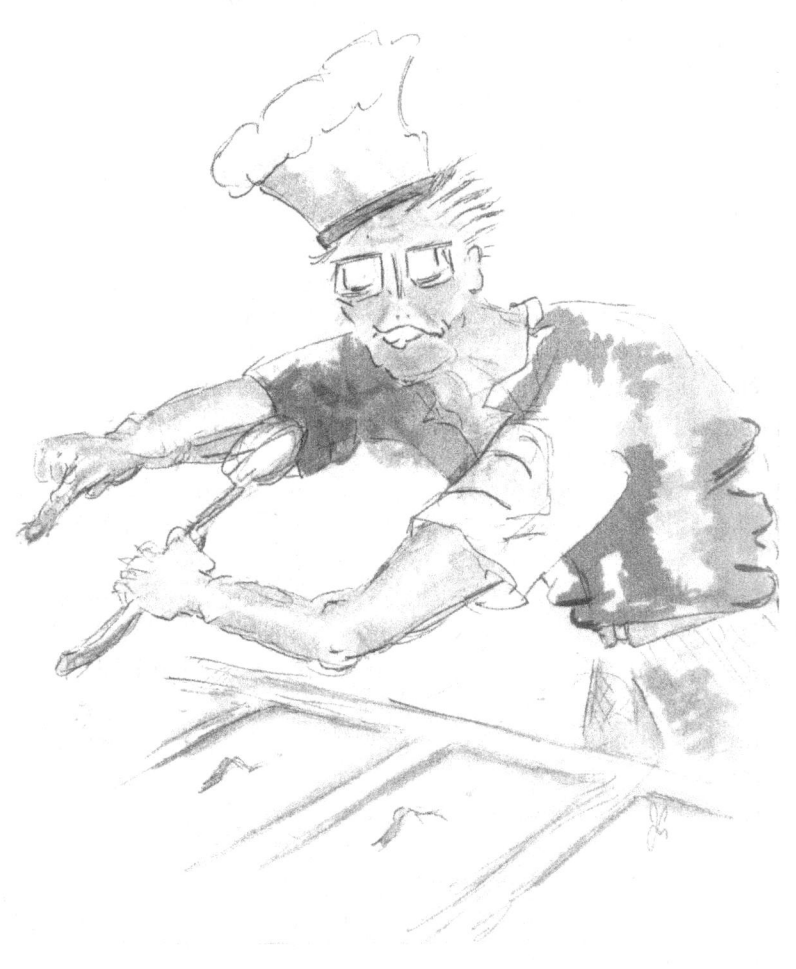

'I'm going to write a book, too – called, 'I had to work with her!'

a nice change from hearing him once say, 'You're brain dead and you've got early Alzheimer's disease...[after a pause] and I mean that in the most caring possible way!'. Fancy calling a person who has had a stroke 'brain dead"!

In spite of Peter (or maybe because of him) the kitchen atmosphere was very supportive and it was a comfortable place to be. For all the hassles the kitchen was home to me. I loved working there and I loved the 'girls'. I got the feeling I was accepted just the way I was. At first I did not realise how kind they were to me but little by little as they told me hilarious stories of how I was in the early days, I got the picture. And they were justifiably proud of the progress I had made.

It seemed that many people were fond of saying to me, 'All you need is confidence'. That was emphatically not so! It was not a matter of confidence: it was a matter of a lack of speech. These people who were well-meaning saw me going round with an air of shyness and unbearable timidity. They probably wanted to shake me. But one cannot be confident without a ready answer. Much of the time although I was aware of the need to respond I could not. It felt as if somebody had taken a cleaver to my brain. I could hear my thoughts 'shouting' in a faraway place but they could not bridge the gap to speech that the cleaver had made.

I felt intuitively that when the gap closed up and the dendrites had regrown, I would get back my former level of confidence.

The three years between my stroke and the time I finished writing this book were among the loneliest years of my life. Three years is a long time for a friendship to last when one side (mine) does not give any input to the relationship. I felt my friends drifting away; doing other things that did not include me. They invited me to a few dinner parties and the odd film and outing. Some forgot my birthday after a while.

However the hard core who did stick around regardless of my condition deserve a medal. At an assertiveness class in April 1989 a woman with a badly damaged back said to the group, 'My friends don't even ask me whether I want to come to this or that. They make up their minds and leave me out.' I remarked, 'I find the same thing'. She said, nastily, 'I'll bet they do, if you can't even communicate with them. It would be far worse than a bad back.' That shook me. I realised something I had been putting out of my conscious thinking, that just because people were being polite about my lack of speech, it did not mean they enjoyed my company. That thought increased my feeling of vulnerability.

I had a dream some time after that incident. It was of a little village in Denmark (in Scandinavia) on the side of a hill. I walked into a gallery with pleasant pictures on the wall and a display of glass ornaments on a table. I picked up a glass ornament and it crumbled in my hand. Looking around I saw that one or two customers had seen me do it and were looking at me. It seemed to me that I had the choice of offering to pay for the damage or making a run for it through the open door. Deciding to pay, I went through a door at the back of the gallery looking for the owner. He was painting. He was tall, slim and wore glasses. He could barely communicate but this fact seemed not to bother him at all. I thought to myself, 'There's an attractive man, even if he can't speak'. I felt better about myself because I had seen him and I felt glad (in the dream) I had not bolted out of the shop.

Some years later while having a glass of wine with Tom I said, 'In case you don't know it, I really appreciate the way you stuck by me when I couldn't get two words straight, couldn't think a coherent thought and my imagination was shot to pieces'.

He thought about it for a moment then said, 'It didn't matter much to me, what you were like; you see you still had the same "essence".'

A little wine and a lot of emotion contributed to more than a bit of a sob about that! Maybe that was what my dream had been trying to tell me.

A great deal of my personality had been lost. I did not realise it for a while but I began to comprehend the full extent of it about eighteen months after the stroke. Along with the lack of imagination, the lack of ideas and the stuttering, I had other difficulties. I found it impossible to make pleasantries, I blurted things out and frightened people I could not think of anything to say and could not initiate conversations. Speech was so difficult that I did not have the concentration and the energy to maintain friendship.

That was the case especially when I had not seen someone for a while and I expected to take up where we left off. I was struggling – as if I were seeing them through a pane of glass, trapped. I think women especially reach out with their emotions but I could not. What I could say to a friend, lacked lustre. I recently read Stephanie Dowrick's book *Intimacy and Solitude* and I realise now that what I lacked was a sense of 'self'. Ms Dowrick (quoting Marie-Louise von Franz) talks of 'self' as 'the solid ground inside oneself'. The 'quicksands' of my mind were not allowing that sense of 'self'. Maybe Ms Dowrick did not intend her words to be taken quite so literally but they were a revelation to me. Perhaps now I was aware of the problem, the brain clicks would get to work on it.

I think that one of the things that made my personality so 'thin' is that my brain seemed to be locked away in a separate compartment away from the speech that came out of my mouth. I knew that somewhere I was receiving messages. I listened to the news and I understood very well what people were saying to me; there was no impairment there. But at the mouth – the mouth is what counts – what I said was my total thought. I might say, 'This house is very nice'. But I had no 'backup' or reference. My mind did not remind me that there were other forms of architecture – houses with a verandah all round, with a mezzanine floor or with a tin roof. That was not available to me.

About two years after the stroke I began to have 'backup' thoughts about 'tin roofs' and ''mezzanine floors' but they were still not connected to speech. Eventually I was able to put these thoughts into speech.

Now people have the impression that I am talking normally (six years later). But they do not know what I am leaving out. And it is that sort of thing that affects friendships. I know the areas that are going to be difficult for me and rather that let that affect my fluency, I subtly leave them out.

I never attempted to explain or describe anything. I would have liked to talk about chemistry and biology to Ben when he was studying but twelve months after the stroke I still was not up to it. It was not until nearly three years after the stroke that I could discuss meiosis (a sort of cell division) with him. It took me a long time and a lot of trial and error before I got to the point but eventually I did it.

Eleven months after the stroke I put an advertisement in a newspaper for a wardrobe and bookcase. The telephone rang, 'You have a bookcase for sale?'

'Yes' I said. This was going to be easy.

'Could you describe it, please?'

'Yes, it's...'. all the thoughts swam in my head at once. It was made of...pine...six foot high (I could not think in metric measurements)...two cupboards...and...how do you describe the vertical bits of wood for records? I was completely silent.

'Well, what's it made of?' the man said impatiently.

'Wood.'

'How high is it?' he said showing signs of exasperation.

'It's...[remember how bad I was with numbers] it's...the height of a door.' I sold it to those people for half as much as I had been asking and threw in the wardrobe as well just so that I would not have to answer the telephone again.

That exercise was a prelude to redesigning Ben's room. Ben was coming home from England at the end of June 1989. I had to work out some 'befores' and 'afters'. Before the carpet went down the ceiling had to be repaired. And after the ceiling was repaired I could paint it and the walls – things like that. I found that with plenty of time to think about it nothing went wrong. Painting the ceiling gave me minor hassles, I lost the feeling in my right arm and leg. That scared me. I took two sleeping pills and cried myself to sleep. But in the morning I was quite all right. It must have been muscle fatigue.

Everyone has the feeling at some time or another that they are missing a word that is just on the tip of their tongue. But the feeling was a bit different for me. One day in June 1989 I spent from ten o'clock in the morning trying to find a word (someone needed it for a crossword) that meant male and female in the same animal. Yvonne came round to see me that evening and she entered into the spirit of the thing by not telling me the answer. I worked out that it began with an H. It was like pulling gently at a word that was attached to a piece of string; teasing away at it and finally landing it. By ten o'clock that night I had it: 'hermaphrodite'!

It was almost as though the dendrites had made the first tentative contacts between my stored thoughts and where the cleaver had made the gap and were linking up to speech. As more and more linked up I was able to recall more and more words.

I had the feeling now that concepts that I thought were lost were coming back to me slowly. It was extremely frustrating. They would fade away like moonshine the moment I tried to pin them down with speech. It was a sensation so fleeting that I hardly knew it was there. But now I was aware of it.

My timidity and shyness became more frustrating as I became more aware of them. The pen and speech are certainly mightier than the sword. My feeling of vulnerability was overwhelming. I was by now almost as strong physically as I used to be but without my speech I was nothing.

As usual as soon as I started to miss a faculty three or four weeks later I had a brain click and what I thought was missing would return. In August 1989 I suddenly found that I could think more quickly than I could speak. And I knew it would only be a matter of time before I would be speaking at the pace of my thoughts.

All this time I was getting better. No one at work ever criticised me (I think that would have been devastating for me). Sandra praised my sandwiches. I was happy. Looking back I think the happy atmosphere of the kitchen did much to restore me.

I do not think I expected to lose empathy the way I did. In November 1989 Yvonne took me to visit some of the stroke patients she was nursing. Although I had some degree of fluency by then I just could not say anything kind to them at all. It was not as if I did not know I was not saying anything reassuring to them; I did. I tried hard but the more I tried the more miserable it made me feel. I quickly became tired from the effort but still I could not find a single word of comfort. I was ashamed of myself and became very depressed about it.

It was much the same thing a few months before when I had lunch with a teaching sister from my old school. She had had a mastectomy and was still very much in shock at the time. Again I tried to say something comforting but I could not and that incident left me depressed as well. I rang her the next day apologising for my lack of feeling. But there was not a thing I could do about it. I did not know when or if that aspect of my personality would ever come back. I am glad to say it did about two years later. But there were fleeting glimpses of it's return before this.

I had a revolutionary thought in October 1989. I thanked Sandra. Suddenly I could see my presence in the kitchen had been trying for my co-workers. Sandra was in the kitchen at the time I had the thought. Much later I wondered if this was a sign of empathy returning. It seemed too that I was more able to admire the babies in the maternity wing.

About this time a stroke patient, with speech problems said to me, 'You are the best'. The comment was prompted by a cup of tea. Remembering my own time in hospital I had asked him if he wanted tea. He said, 'Yes'. And it was clear to me from my own experience and by the pained look on his face that he was simply echoing me and he really wanted something else. I waited until 'tea' went out of his mind with a feat of concentration much like my own in the early days. Finally he said, 'Coffee'.

By September 1989 I was really very tired and decided to ask Ms McIntosh for some annual leave. The day before I saw her I had worked out what I wanted to say. It was enormously difficult for me to think of the right thing to say. That was another thing that made me seem to lack 'confidence'. A lot of the things that pass for common courtesy were things I had to relearn.

Nothing seemed right. I knew I had to get the words 'annual leave' and 'two weeks' in there somewhere. I knew also that Ms McIntosh did not have to grant holidays before an employee had been there a year; it was a privilege. I had been at the job for seven months.

I had the request in my mind as I went in to her office. 'Good morning, Jennifer. What can I do for you?'

Of course I forgot the courtesy, 'Good morning, Matron'. (I called Ms McIntosh 'Matron' because it was easier for me.) I just said, 'Good morning' – and that promptly pushed the rest of what I wanted to say out of my mind.

After closing the door I rushed forward leaned my two hands of her desk (in what I imagine was quite a threatening manner) and blurted out, 'Could I have the holidays due to me?'.

If Ms McIntosh was taken aback, she did not show it. And thank goodness she did not. I felt bad enough already. The next day I apologised for the way in which I had asked for my holiday. She said that they were all intrigued by my progress and not to worry about it.

The next day I made an appointment to see Isobel, my new speech pathologist. Isobel proved to be very helpful. She spotted the trouble at once: 'It's your sociotypical phrasing' she said. I felt relieved that there was a word to describe my condition, but what did it mean and could it be cured?

She said, 'Apart from the way you dress, your body language and the first words you utter, make an impact. They tell the other person whether you come aggressively or as a friend.' We worked on strategies for explaining and describing things and for initiating conversations, which was another weakness. And we talked about ideas. In order to have ideas you have to have the words (the vocabulary) to express the concept. During the illness I felt constantly upset that I did not have words. I could not recall or retain information and consequently ideas were not easily accessible; they were hidden, fuzzy.

Isobel suggested I go for assertiveness training. I did not really benefit from that though. I gave up after a few sessions believing that I could not be assertive without words or the ability to express ideas.

The symptoms that were the legacy of the stroke gradually improved (even without the more dramatic help of the brain clicks) throughout 1989 and 1990. One day in early 1989 quite by chance I picked up a Jeffery Archer novel and found I could read it! I thought at first that I had had a brain click so I seized *Berlin Game* (the one I had had all the trouble with) and tried that too but Len Deighton's sentence structure was still too complex for me. It was not until September 1989 after a brain click that I could read *Berlin Game* with any real understanding. But now I had hope. If there was one book I could read there must be more. I discovered in time that I could read Helen MacInnes, Barbara Erskine (*Lady of Hay*) and Arthur Hailey.

I had a bad habit of staring at people. After a brain click in October 1989 that habit disappeared. Soon after my arithmetic improved. I was very glad when my emotional reaction to music returned, the result of a brain click in June 1990. One evening driving down the freeway I turned on the radio to find the song 'Love is Blue' playing. I associated that song with a very happy time in my life. The old feelings came back just as they used to! When I had heard it earlier in the illness I knew intuitively the feelings it was supposed to have engendered on hearing it, but it did not; it just left me numb. I felt that as a huge loss.

On the debit side I was at times still feeling gauche, blurting things out and even blushing and it was still very difficult for me to initiate a conversation. I missed not being able to talk to people in shops about trivial things like the weather.

I started to put in my diary estimations of my speech recovery compared to how it was in the days before I had the stroke. Eighty per cent I wrote one year after the stroke; seventy-five per cent six months later; fifty percent six months after that. The decreasing figures only go to prove I did not know at the time how bad I was. I seemed to get a worse score the more enlightened I became. Maybe when I get to twenty per cent of what I thought I was like before, I'll be speaking quite well.

Gradually my intolerance receded and I did not fly off the handle as often as I did before. I got along better at work and was able to join in the conversations. People began to notice I had more of a sense of humour.

I found myself shouting out as other people would do. I knew now that if I shouted from one end of the kitchen, 'There's milk in the fridge!'. I could be confident that I would not stop half-way through it because I had forgotten what I was saying. It was all wonderfully liberating.

Around this time my perceptive friend Jasmine said, 'You are a bit like a computer, you have length and width but certain areas weren't accessible until now. Now you are developing depth.'

However there were times when I realised very clearly how far I still had to go. On a visit to Dr B in January 1990 I told him that Ms McIntosh had another job for me when I felt ready to tackle it. I visualised the possible job. I believed I could be a ward assistant in time when I could answer the telephone without dread. Or perhaps it was in the office? I saw myself sitting down in a chair in the office. I was wearing the red, white and black of the office staff and I was distributing letters and flowers to the patients. I looked at Dr B and smiled, feeling pleased with myself. He said, 'Well?'. And I realised what I had been doing. I had been just thinking it. How many other people had I 'explained' things to and just thought them?

I wondered how the other people from the Outward Bound Group were getting on. It was June 1990 and I had not seen them since I had started work eighteen months before. I asked Chris, the group's speech pathologist to have lunch with me. She told me Jean was painting again and Yvonne had a voluntary job with Meals-on-Wheels. All the group members were speaking better now.

It was not until April 1990 that I had a brain click that transformed me overnight from a hesitant speaker (choosing carefully what was said) to a person willing to start a sentence with the hope that it would come out all right in the end.

As I became more fluent my confidence rose. My writing improved again. It was a far cry from when I could not even write my signature. That loss seemed strange to me – I thought my signature would have been so deeply ingrained into my personality that I would never forget it. As a result of my fluency improving, I was a 'whizz' on the telephone – comparatively!

One of the most enlightening moments for me was in August 1990 when I started to remember more of my background. Before then I could remember the things that had happened during the previous year or so in the right order. But although earlier events – even from as far back as twenty years – were recalled, there were no 'steps' of memory. For example I would remember working in a laboratory in Bristol in the early 1970's and at another time remember walking in the corridor of a Canberra hospital when I worked there three years previously but without being able to put the two events on separate memory 'steps'. I could not separate the two memories. When you cannot put memories into sequence you lose a lot of colour from life. Suddenly for me the colour came back with my properly sequenced memories.

People would say to me, 'You must feel very frustrated'. It made me wonder why I did not at once agree with them and I realised that were using the wrong word for what I was in fact feeling. I could not correct them then because I myself could not express the feeling with any clarity. Loss of speech, and the thoughts that go with it, is so catastrophic that 'frustration' does not go nearly far enough to describe it. It is total loss. I think when people use the word 'frustration', they really have in mind the inability to get words out. But it is much more than that. I was aware of the fragmentation of my brain – the emotions, body language and thoughts that were all cut off and out of my reach. I could reach some of them but not all of them together, as I needed to do for normal speech. No, 'frustration' definitely is not the word. If that was all it was I could have become angry and some of the 'frustration' would most likely have disappeared. To paraphrase Wordsworth, mine was a grief 'too deep for tears'.

CHAPTER FOURTEEN

Stretching the Brain

Almost from the moment Ben set foot back on home ground he was urging me to go swimming. He set out at five-thirty in the morning to go to the wretched pool. There was no way I was going to do that. I did not swim well, only breaststroke – what is more I did not like swimming much.

Of course the day came when I agreed to go with him. I could see that unless I tried it, Ben would be justified in calling me a 'wimp'. And I was glad that he cared so much about my rehabilitation. Ben went with me that first time. It was midwinter and the pool was open air but heated. 'How heated?' I wanted to know. It was about ten in the morning and a watery sun was shining. If it were not for the fact that I had to go in the pool it would have been a lovely day.

The pool was beautifully warm, a little fresh when I came out but there was a hot shower. I swam three times a week from then on. I worked up from four laps of breast stroke to eight. I felt if I tried to push myself to do any more I would not come swimming at all, so I stayed at eight. I had always been a believer in the saying 'A fit mind in a fit body'. Now was my chance to see if it was true – the hard way.

I thought of the treatment that is given to children with cerebral palsy. Volunteers come in relays to exercise their arms and legs for up to eight hours a day. Rosemary, when she saw I had taken up swimming remembered that movement of the arms is thought to be especially good for stimulating the brain. I was glad to hear it but apart from that I liked swimming now and it did remarkable things for my speech. So I continued.

I did other things to further my speech. Reading seemed to help. I had progressed from a page or two at a time to one or two chapters. It was still a lot of concentration for me particularly when I had to work. I usually walked ten to twenty minutes a day. Isobel, my speech pathologist sent me to relaxation classes and I found them beneficial too.

I have not mentioned much about my physical progress. Fortunately the physical damage caused by the stroke was insignificant compared with the damage to my speech. Nevertheless it was there.

After the stroke my eyes were blurred for about seven weeks. And it took about a week to get the feeling back in my right hand sufficient for me to hold a knife. I dragged my right foot when I was allowed out of bed.

I did not really notice these things much when they were lost, I noticed them more when they disappeared. For example about twelve months after the stroke my posture improved a little. But I still could not walk comfortably and I did not swing my right arm as I walked. Years later I happened to mention this to Rod. He said with alacrity, 'Yes, you looked like a gorilla with your arms dangling around your knees, when you first arrived!'. Surprisingly I did not mind the observation. My co-workers including Rod accepted me, illness and all and their attitude made me feel I fitted in and gave me a sense of security.

My poor posture was hurting my back and I had never had trouble with my back before the stroke. At first I thought it was pushing the hot box that was causing my back pain and I put up with it because I did not want anything to interfere with my job. But it was not that, I think it was not being at ease with my body so the muscles were tense and rigid.

And then in January 1990 I had a brain click and my posture, as well as my speech improved again. I noticed that my right foot no longer scraped the floor (I had pulled the sole off an expensive pair of shoes once in this way) and I had no more back trouble. I started swinging my right arm. These were all faculties I was not aware I had lost, until they were returned.

Someone told me about Feldenkrais, which is described as 'awareness through movement...good for posture and flexibility'. I thought it sounded just the thing for me so I went along to an introductory lesson. It consists of very gentle, soothing exercises. I liked it a lot but I could not get to any more classes which were held during the day while I was working.

One thing that can be said in favour of my stroke is that I felt quite well physically after the initial damage. From then on I got better. I was not troubled by feelings of nausea or headaches at all, several people were surprised at how well I looked. I did not have anything to stop me progressing except the exhaustion due to concentrating. But I found that the more

I pushed myself the easier it became to push back the fatigue of concentration. I could carry on with the same thing a little longer the next day.

Writing this book has been of enormous benefit, very therapeutic. I had kept a diary for a number of years before my illness and as soon as I was able I began writing in it again. It has been invaluable particularly for plotting the brain clicks. When I started to write the book about eighteen months after the stroke, how I had to concentrate even to write one paragraph! It would take me over an hour and then I would have to sleep. Gradually over the next six months I crept up to almost a page in two hours. All the time my concentration got better. Vonny, my neighbour would call and over a cup of coffee I would give her the next page of my manuscript to read. She was always very encouraging and urged me to continue.

I reminded myself that at the time of my stroke nobody could find me a book about a stroke affecting the speech centres. I would have liked to have known how other people coped with the same thing. That (and the fact that even friends did not really understand my predicament) is when I promised myself that, should I be fortunate enough to recover I would write about what had happened to me. Writing the book affected other areas too. My reading improved and so did my speech so I was convinced that I was doing the right thing.

Another way of pushing myself was the courses and exercise I embarked on. The woodwork, typing and swimming all helped my speech. Later I became more ambitious and went on a weekend course called 'Anger: Flame of Life'. That is when I realised, to my horror that I was more or less devoid of emotion. And to make matters worse I had continued to think that one day I would be able to write romance novels! My imagination did not function at all well either. The course instructor (a psychologist) urged us to, 'Think of one person who did something bad to you and with whom you feel anger'. Soon everyone was scribbling away with crayons on pieces of paper; some were down on the floor so fully had they entered into the spirit of the thing. I sat bolt upright on my chair, gnawing my pencil and metaphorically scratching my head. I could not think of anyone (I can now!). The instructor's verdict: 'You are very controlled, Jenny'. I used to be quite emotional.

Dr B said 'word processing' would improve my fluency. I was to pick any letter of the alphabet, say S, and in five minutes write down as many three (and over) - syllable words beginning with S that I could think of – I could use a dictionary to check my list. This exercise improved my fluency considerably. When Dr B first suggested it to me in his office (two and a half years after the stroke) I was lucky to think of two words. As I got used to it I began to get six or seven words and within a few weeks I was quite good at it.

It seemed anything that made me tired from concentration was good for me. When I had visited Ben in England part of my son's idea of entertaining his mother was to let her join in his Russian lessons. Ben had previously taught himself German from a book and tapes and was now embarking on Russian, my visit coincided with the lessons. I found it amusing. I could barely speak English, let alone Russian! At that time I did not realise the benefit of tiring myself so I let the lessons lapse after I came back to Perth. But they were very strenuous: ten minutes of a Russian lesson was worth an hour of typing! I read that the brain in older people (seventy years and older), can be stimulated by learning new things. The article described 'an explosion of neuron activity' as a result of learning a foreign language.

I do not think it matters what sport, occupation or study is used to 'stretch' the brain and its concentration, as long as it is done every day.

I feel work was probably the biggest factor in my recovery especially living on my own as I do and I am very grateful to have been given the opportunity by Colleen McIntosh to work so soon after my stroke. Without the work I may not have been so aware of what I have called brain clicks. I had to concentrate continuously at first and although it made me tired I believe it hastened the phenomena of brain clicks.

People were very patient and understanding at the hospital and this allowed me slowly to regain my confidence. After I had just started work, Yvonne not wanting me to be too upset if I was fired said, 'Consider this as a 'disposable' job just to get you into the swing of things again'. That was sound advice and fortunately I did not have to change my job.

People talked in the breaks between work and just listening to them brought back long-buried conversational habits, so by the time I was ready to say something it was not a major trauma, it seemed natural.

I found I just had to suffer my timidity. If I had to put my loss of faculties into the order of most regretted I would put 'not being able to read' first, then 'timidity' second, 'loss of humour' third, followed by 'loss of imagination and emotions'. Strangely actual 'loss of speech' ranks in my mind below these faculties.

Those schoolgirl fears about stroke that had beset me all those years ago were not so far wrong as it happens. It is a rotten thing to suffer a stroke. It was the thought of being utterly dependent on somebody else that would send me into a tailspin. In those days I thought of a stroke purely in terms of paralysis. By good luck I was largely spared that aspect of stroke. But I was not spared the dependence on other people. When I lost my speech I became dependent upon others for understanding. If other people chose not to be patient while I stumbled and stammered about I could not do anything about it.

My friends and Ben were wonderful and they steadfastly did not let me down, even though mine was the first stroke or serious illness of any kind among them. It must have been very hard for them not knowing what was going to happen and if I would get better or not.

I was grumbling at Ben one day and the conversation was not going my way so I started to shout. Soon my speech ran together. I was breathing hard and went red in the face. 'Look what you've done!', I yelled. 'It's enough to give me another stroke.' I stopped short of saying, 'And you'll miss me when I'm gone'. Ben looked at me. 'Don't you put that emotional blackmail on me, Mum' he said firmly and he opened the door and went out. I never tried that again.

Recently we happened to have in the hospital a patient, called Bob who had had a stroke and completely lost his speech. I went into his room to offer him a supper-time drink from my trolley. He gave me a lovely smile and gestured meaninglessly. Eventually he picked up a card from the table which said, 'NO'. It took me back to my days in hospital especially the meaningless gestures. I could take things in very nicely (at that stage) but could not get them out again, I could not communicate. What must it have been like for my friends who saw me like that?

Peter had borrowed a newspaper from Bob and he asked me to take it back to him. Hoping that he, like me, could understand perfectly well I said to him, 'I had a stoke like the one you had'. I pointed to the left-hand side of my head and my right arm which I held limply to resemble paralysis. He was delighted and smiled. But I thought to myself how disorientating it was to talk to him and not know for sure that he understood. It was a humbling experience. That was how my friends had felt; I knew I could make sense of every word they spoke to me but how could they be sure? Rosemary and Tom (when he returned from his trip abroad) saw me most days and never let me know by so much as a glance what they really felt about my chances if full recovery.

Bob could not tell me to put the newspaper on the chair behind me. He waved his hands about and his eyes filled with tears (just as mine had at every minor frustration) as I put it on the table in front of him. I put my hand on his arm and said he would soon be better – just look at me, I was better now! He smiled again. Later I had to take him a banana sandwich. Irreverently I wondered how the sister who ordered it had managed to establish that that was what he wanted. It was not on the menu. I took the sandwich in to Bob and it was indeed what he wanted. Unwrapping the sandwich I asked him if he would like another cup of coffee. He put his hand firmly over his cup. It was an abrupt movement and I was momentarily a little taken aback by it. But I had been very abrupt in the early stages too so why should I be surprised? I realised my friends and relatives had had to put up with all sorts of inappropriate behaviour from me.

I talked to Bob some more. I said waving my arms about, 'Even out gestures are meaningless, aren't they?' He was delighted with that observation, he was beaming and tearful at the same time. And I went smiling – and tearful – back to the kitchen.

CHAPTER FIFTEEN

Twenty-Three Years Later

Two decades have passed since I wrote my book and I am now living in semi-retirement, playing golf and writing.

While I was still working at South Perth Hospital I became interested in Reflexology and went to a weekend course. Reflexology is the 'application of alternating pressure to the feet and hands'. The reflex areas on the feet and hands of the organs, glands and tissues were mapped by the Egyptians and Chinese more than 2500 BC. If my goals in life had to change, then I might try this. Reflexology had several things to recommend it. It was something I could do that did not involve me in talking, I liked doing it and people seemed to benefit from my ministrations. I did a two year course after the weekend introductory course at the West Australian School of Reflexology. I thought seriously about setting up in business but one thing I am not is a businesswoman: the idea fell through. However I benefited from the course unexpectedly. Working with my hands was immensely good for the brain. As I have mentioned before, the workings of the hand takes up a rather large area in the brain. The extra stimulation of the hand movement seemed to speed up the process of getting my speech back.

In spite of the illness, I was fortunate enough to slip into a relationship with a new boyfriend, someone I did not know before I had the stroke. If he was going to accept me he would do so without the baggage of knowing what I was like before the illness. He was humorous, practical and loving, not a talkative man and did not expect me to be either!

I was in two minds as to whether it would have been better to have had a partner to help me through the trauma or not. I decided I was glad after all that I was on my own. It was my biggest fear that several of my friends would leave me. So how much worse would it have been to have a partner leave? I have been through a divorce where I spent a year or two afterwards feeling like one half of a whole person. Two or three people in the speech pathology classes had had just that happen to them: a partner leave them. It must have been devastating for them to have lost partners and had a stroke as well.

I saw my friend quite regularly but not every day. I do not believe it would have lasted very long, with the burden of my 'thin' personality and speech problems. Although I would have liked to see more of him I was realistic enough to know that it would have been a struggle for me and would have fired up my feelings of inadequacy. To say nothing of his feelings about the matter. He was always constant, never left me wondering when

I would be seeing him again. That aspect of the friendship was doubly important in my case where I needed to spend all my energies on the process of getting well again, rather than worry about losing him as a friend. He had inevitably come to mean a lot to me by that time.

I continued to work at South Perth Community Hospital for another year until Colleen McIntosh, who had been so understanding and kind to me, retired. Peter, Rod and Sandra were restless and looking for change and the 'world order' in my cosy kitchen was threatening to come to an end. Besides, I had been in my comfort zone long enough – time to try something new.

My application for a job as a phlebotomist (blood-taking) was successful. I had taken plenty of blood in my years in medical science. My practical experiences with the screwdriver and rolling serviettes had given me the dexterity I needed for phlebotomy again and I enjoyed the one-on-one contact with patients in the Medical Centres I worked in.

The learning curve for me was to make people feel comfortable. A bit of empathy was needed, especially with children. I still do phlebotomy in a part-time capacity and I really enjoy chatting to people! Nowadays I never have to tell people I have had a stroke unless I have a person visit me who is in the same predicament – then I cannot resist it.

Yvonne and I joined a Romance Writers group run by Anna Jacobs. Anna was very generous with her advice and supportive criticism. We had a fruitful time and learnt a lot about the art of writing. I found I could write a lot better than I could talk. The ideas and imagination were still missing but slowly getting better.

The government cut contact time, for speech pathologists running group therapy, from once a week to once a fortnight.

Our group wanted to go on having weekly meetings and Melita Brown, with the group's approval, arranged that I should run it. It was not very successful. I fretted over the task and stumbled over words. I do not think anyone enjoyed it much, particularly me.

Then I rather foolishly agreed to teach a course in Medical Terminology for medical receptionists at CYSS. Yvonne had been teaching it but she wanted to go to another job and she thought of me. By the middle of the first session I suddenly burst into tears and said, 'I love human biology and I am sorry I am not doing this subject any justice. I'll leave and you can have someone else who can teach it properly'. They were lovely young women, they persuaded me to stay and they taught themselves with a minimum of help from me. I could answer questions pretty well by that time but could not deliver a set speech. They worked in little groups among themselves and everybody passed the required test at the end!

That was definitely the end of teaching for me! Reflexology or phlebotomy were beginning to look more and more attractive.

One positive thing the stroke did for me was to make me self-reliant. Previously I was a bit anxious and not happy unless there were people around me. In the four years of almost total isolation after the illness, I learned to really like and appreciate my own company. I must have discovered, at last, the sense of 'self 'that Stephanie Dowrick talks about in her book *Intimacy & Solitude*.

My son Ben became a general practitioner and married Amanda who is warm and funny, with a biting wit – my kind of person.

I asked Dr Carroll how bad my stroke really was. He said, on a scale of one to ten it was a nine - yet he never put a limit on my recovery. Several people in the speech therapy groups I have attended have had a limitations thrust on them by members of the medical profession. They are convinced they will only recover up to two years. 'After two years', they say, 'one does not recover any further.' That sort of statement affects the relatives and friends, as well as the patient. Luckily for me, Dr Carroll emphatically does not believe that one only recovers for two years. I think when people say patients will not recover much after that time, they are forgetting an important thing. The *obvious* recovery that people around you are aware of is made in about two years. But the real recovery that matters to the person themselves is an ongoing internal process. Enjoyment of more and more of life, music, humour, a sense of your own history - these are things that make you more secure. Things like that do not show on the outside of a person.

If Bill Carroll had told me I would only recover for two years, then that would have been that. I doubt if I would have had the fulfilling life I enjoy today. At that time I was very suggestible to the words of Bill Carroll. Instead he told me, 'We must not underestimate the long-term ability of the human brain to recover.' And I believed him.

EPILOGUE

The following is a list of the major events and milestones in my progress after the stroke, including the brain clicks [designated BC's] of which I was aware. Although I did not become aware of BC's until January 1989 there were breakthroughs before this that would almost certainly have been the result of a BC.

After each BC my speech, fluency and writing usually improved but these are not necessarily described.

I hope my experiences may help another stroke patient somewhere.

JULY 1988
6	Stroke; admitted to QE11. Unable to speak for six days
12	Grunting noises
13	Sounds
20	Tried to write sentence (with left hand), very tiring
21	Tried to read, managed a sentence or two 23-24 Allowed out of hospital (Rosemary and Allen's house) for weekend
27	Angiogram

AUGUST 1988
4	Allowed out of hospital (shopping with Duncan)
8	Moved from QE11 to Shenton Park
26	BC Blurriness gone from right eye
27-28	Allowed out of hospital (Margaret's house) for weekend BC Read magazine it started to make sense

SEPTEMBER 1988
- 2   Discharged from hospital
- 16   First Outward Bound Group meeting

OCTOBER 1988
- 13   BC Writing easier
- 14   BC Told one-word joke; handwriting improved; speaking more freely
- 17   Began typing course (until 28/10/88). Through course, concentration improved

NOVEMBER 1988
- 7   Began woodwork course (until trip in December). Through course, coordination improved
- 22   Played golf again

DECEMBER 1988
- 3   Left Perth to fly to London via Singapore (one night stopover)
- 9   Russian lesson with Ben; improvement in writing thoughts

JANUARY 1989
- 10   Became aware that BC's made the world seem more expansive and I felt more in tune with it
- 18   Arrived back in Perth

FEBRUARY 1989
- 7   Started job in hospital

APRIL 1989
- 7   BC Faster and more organised at work; more chatty; less tired
- 17   BC Much faster at work; found myself chatting to a stroke patient

MAY 1989

1   BC Faster at work; not as timid; beginning to say things that are uncensored

5   BC breakthrough in speech; words come to me more easily; some ideas; repartee

29   BC Beginning to get back a rudimentary sense of humour; answer a patient's question without hesitation

JUNE 1989

2   BC More fluent

17   BC Smiled a little more; able to crack an aspirin tablet down the centre; posture improving

20   BC Felt that concepts that I thought were lost to me were just around the corner

JULY 1989

24   Called Shirley a bitch – considered my recovery had begun

25   Eyelids twitching (nerves regenerating)

AUGUST 1989

18   BC I could think faster than I could speak – it was a start

SEPTEMBER 1989

18   BC Able to read Len Deighton's *Berlin Game* very slowly and understand it

OCTOBER 1989

2   BC Thanked Sandra for her kindness – new thing to find the words to express what I felt

20   BC Able to think of more things to say but I did not like to vocalise them; afraid of boring people with my hesitancy. No longer stared at people as much

26	BC Counting better. Still found it difficult to initiate a conversation; found things to say but not quickly enough. Humming recognisable tunes; yelling out confidently in the kitchen; talking more fluently

NOVEMBER 1989

12	BC Dramatic improvement in speech; occurred after John had taken me to a charismatic meeting at the Redemptorist Monastery in Perth. Prayers seemed to help

JANUARY 1990

9	BC Right arm (which had previously remained limp) swung when I walked; no longer caught my right foot on the floor; muscles no longer tense and rigid

FEBRUARY 1990

18	Started writing book

APRIL 1990

25	BC Breakthrough in speech; willing to start a sentence now with the hope it would come out all right in the end

MAY1990

8	BC Faster at work; joining in conversations
26	BC Joined in the fun at work; made comical remarks

JUNE 1990

9	BC My emotional interest in music restored; I could sing in tune too; fluency and confidence improved

JULY 1990

21	BC Handwriting improved; much better at

talking on the telephone (no longer needed to write down what I wanted to say)

AUGUST 1990

   1   BC Remembered past events in sequence

  25   BC Told Peter a joke

OCTOBER 1990

   6   BC Eyesight improved; walking no longer 'wooden'

NOVEMBER 1990

   6   BC Still had difficulty explaining things but willing to try now

FEBRUARY 1991

  21   Started 'word processing' exercise with Dr B – this helped enormously

MARCH 1991

  10   BC Answered back to people without hesitation; handwriting improved

APRIL 1991

   2   BC Discussed meiosis (cell division) with Ben

MAY 1991

   6   Finished writing book

The brain clicks tailed off towards the end of 1991 but when massive new insights were needed they were still present. The last distinct brain click I noticed was in May 1993.

It is nearly six years since I had the stroke and my life has changed. The changes have not necessarily been all for the worse but life is certainly different. I earn less money than I did as a medical scientist or as a teacher. Where I work now is relatively stress free and I do not take my work home with me. I enjoy working with my colleagues. And I have more time to devote to friends and family and for just relaxing.

I wonder now why I did not think of following a low-cholesterol diet before I was ill but I probably would not have had the discipline to maintain it. I still occasionally go on a chocolate binge but I stick to the diet apart from that. I feel better on the diet and my skin and hair have improved. Fruit and fish for me are the way to go.

Ron Saw mentions in his book the importance of keeping in touch with a neurologist. I continue to see Dr B the specialist neurologist who was responsible for my care. With my speech disorder I also keep in touch with Melita Brown. Speech pathologists do not just stop at getting you to make the word sounds; they work with you until you are satisfied that you are really on the right track to recovery. At present I am one of a group of five people who attend a speech therapy group run by Melita at Bentley Hospital. Even at this stage (in 1994) it is well worth it; a clever speech pathologist makes a vast difference to fluency and in particular awareness of everyday life.

Now most people do not realise that I have had a stroke. At most, some of them think I have a slight stutter. I am content with the amount of personality and imagination that has returned to me. At this stage I can see that I would be ready to resume some sort of teaching – perhaps tutoring – at some later date. Or I may even try and write that romance novel.

The '97.86 per cent of normal' that Dr B promised me in QE11 now looks eminently possible.

FURTHER READING

SPEECH STROKE

Dahlberg, Charles Clay, *Stroke: A Doctor's Personal Story of His Recovery*, 1st edn, Norton, New York, c. 1977

Griffith, V.C. *A Stroke in the Family*, Dell Publishing Co. Inc., New York, 1970

Isted, Charles R., *Learning to Speak Again After a Stroke*, King's Fund Publishing Office, London, 1979

Law, Diana, *Living After a Stroke*, Souvenir Press (Educational and Academic) Ltd, London, 1980

Owen, William, *The Road Back: A Stroke Victim's Recovery*, Little Hills Press, Crow's Nest (NSW), 1993

Ritchie, Douglas, *A Diary of Recovery*, Faber and Faber, London, 1960

RELATED SUBJECTS

Dowrick, Stephanie, *Intimacy & Solitude*, Random House, 1991

Hewson, Lorna, *When Half is Whole: My Recovery from Stroke*, Dove Communications, Blackburn (Vic.) 1988

Hewson, Lorna, *Stroke: A Family Affair*, Collins Dove, Blackburn (Vic.) 1988

Hodgins, E., *Episode: - A Report on the Accident Inside My Skull*, Victor Gollancz Ltd, London, 1964

Langton Hewer, R., and Wade, D.T., *Stroke: A Practical Guide Towards Recovery*, Methuen Australia, North Ryde (NSW), 1986

Rose, Frank Clifford, and Capildeo, R., *Stroke: The Facts*, Oxford University Press, New York, 1981

Sacks, Oliver, *Seeing Voices*, Picador by Pan Books, London, 1990

Saw, Ron, *Stroke – And How I Survived It*, Penguin, Ringwood (Vic.), 1985

Sessler, Tom, *Stroke: How to Prevent It, How to Survive It*, Prentice Hall, Englewood Cliffs (NJ), 1981

Smith, Tom, *Coping With Strokes*, Sheldon Press, London, 1991

Styron, William, *Darkness Visible: a Memoir of Madness*, Random House Inc., 1989

Thomas, D.J., *Strokes and Their Prevention*, Equation, in association with the British Medical Association, Wellingborough, 1988

Wentworth, Sally, *Cage of Ice*, Mills and Boon, 1987

ABOUT THE AUTHOR

Jennifer Gordon was born in Nottingham England. After obtaining an honours degree in agricultural science at the University of Nottingham, she emigrated to Australia and worked as a research assistant.

Jennifer became a medical scientist, working at Canberra Community Hospital, before marrying and returning to England. With her son, Benjamin she re-emigrated to Australia and worked in Darwin Hospital before settling in Perth and undertaking a Diploma of Education. She subsequently taught science in high schools, a college of advanced education and medical science at Curtin University of Technology.

Jennifer lives in Mandurah, near Perth accompanied by Jericho, (Maggie, and Hiraeth's successor).

www.ingramcontent.com/pod-product-compliance
Lightning Source LLC
Chambersburg PA
CBHW071502040426
42444CB00008B/1457